Diabetic Meals

In 30 Minutes—Or Less!

2nd Edition

Robyn Webb

Talk to your healthcare provider
about your specific dietary restrictions.

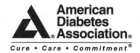

American Diabetes Association.

Cure • Care • Commitment®

Director, Book Publishing, John Fedor; *Associate Director, Consumer Books,* Robert Anthony; *Managing Editor, Book Publishing,* Abe Ogden; *Editor,* Greg Guthrie; *Production Manager,* Melissa Sprott; *Composition,* American Diabetes Association; *Cover Design,* Koncept, Inc.; *Printer,* Worzalla Publishing Co.

Printed in the United States of America

3 5 7 9 10 8 6 4

The suggestions and information contained in this publication are generally consistent with the Clinical Practice Recommendations and other policies of the American Diabetes Association, but they do not represent the policy or position of the Association or any of its boards or committees. Reasonable steps have been taken to ensure the accuracy of the information presented. However, the American Diabetes Association cannot ensure the safety or efficacy of any product or service described in this publication. Individuals are advised to consult a physician or other appropriate health care professional before undertaking any diet or exercise program or taking any medication referred to in this publication. Professionals must use and apply their own professional judgment, experience, and training and should not rely solely on the information contained in this publication before prescribing any diet, exercise, or medication. The American Diabetes Association—its officers, directors, employees, volunteers, and members—assumes no responsibility or liability for personal or other injury, loss, or damage that may result from the suggestions or information in this publication.

⊗ The paper in this publication meets the requirements of the ANSI Standard Z39.48-1992 (permanence of paper).

ADA titles may be purchased for business or promotional use or for special sales. To purchase this book in large quantities, or for custom editions of this book with your logo, contact Lee Romano Sequeira, Special Sales & Promotions, at the address below, or at LRomano@diabetes.org or 703-299-2046.

American Diabetes Association
1701 North Beauregard Street
Alexandria, Virginia 22311

Library of Congress Cataloging-in-Publication Data
Webb, Robyn.
 Diabetic meals in 30 minutes--or less! / Robyn Webb. -- 2nd ed.
   p. cm.
 Includes bibliographical references and index.
 ISBN-13: 978-1-58040-265-1 (alk. paper)
 1. Diabetes--Diet therapy--Recipes. I. Title. II. Title: Diabetic meals in thirty minutes-- or less.

RC662.W355 2006
641.5'6314--dc22

2006017113

*This book is lovingly dedicated to my mother
Ruth, whose own challenges inspire me
and others around her every day.*

CONTENTS

FOREWORD

All too often, I've overheard people who are just diagnosed with diabetes saying that they can't eat what they like anymore. Suddenly, it seems that just discovering you have this disease means that words like "flavor," "savor," and "taste" can no longer apply to life. Nothing could be further from the truth. In fact, in some ways, people who are living with diabetes can discover new and exciting recipes while trying to meet their dietary requirements.

This is not to say that a healthy diabetes diet lets you eat whatever you want, whenever you want. Part of the reason for the increasing rates of obesity and diabetes in the United States comes from our high-fat, high-calorie diets. No doubt you've heard about this epidemic on the news, in the papers, or just from discussions happening around you. So, you'll still be eating differently from how you did before you were diagnosed with diabetes. However, by simply adopting a healthy eating meal plan and adding some exercise to your daily routine, you'll still be able to enjoy diverse, satisfying meals much like the ones you loved so much before your diagnosis.

For 10 years now, Robyn Webb's *Diabetic Meals in 30 Minutes—Or Less!* has helped people with diabetes walk down the new and exciting path of healthy eating. She's even shown us how to incorporate diabetes-friendly recipes into our busy 21st-century diets. It is possible to have a tasty meal ready to eat in 30 minutes, and all it requires is a little forethought and organization. With this kind of helpful guidance, I think you'll find the transition to healthier eating easier, more manageable, and less intimidating.

So let Robyn Webb show you how to prepare quick, tasty, and healthy recipes with this, the revised second edition of her bestselling cookbook for the American Diabetes Association.

Robert A. Rizza, MD
President, Medicine and Science
American Diabetes Association

Preface to the Second Edition

Ten years ago, when *Diabetic Meals in 30 Minutes—or Less!* was first published, the world was a busy place. Today, "busy" is a mild way to describe our frantic, hurried daily lives. The need for quick, convenient healthy food has never been more critical. With the sad statistics of the ever increasing number of people diagnosed with diabetes, healthy eating is not just a wise lifestyle choice, it may also save your life.

These days, it's simply too risky to base your health on food prepared outside your own kitchen. With the ideas in this book, you'll be surprised to see how easy it is to prepare healthy food quickly and with little effort. Plus, you'll get to have great-tasting meals at home, meaning more money in your pocket. The ideas at the beginning of the book will help you to get organized, which is the chief component in the "war" on time. You can't be efficient if you aren't organized, but by learning just a few time-saving tricks, you will keep your kitchen workspace streamlined and efficient.

This book still contains all of the favorite and familiar foods that you and your family enjoy. You'll find that with just a little variation, you'll never be bored with healthy eating. And even though people with diabetes have to adhere to pretty specific dietary guidelines, the first priority here is flavor. Fresh herbs, rich spices, and aromatic vegetables will replace the excess fat, sugars, and sodium that were making your diet unhealthy. There is no reason to suffer from bland meals when you can enjoy ones that are tasty and good for you, too.

Food is one of life's greatest pleasures. Even though having diabetes means that eating must be more carefully experienced, that doesn't mean that we can't continue to gain pleasure from it. All of us should be able to embrace—rather than avoid—our meals and the idea of eating. By using these time-tested recipes, I hope you will all continue to enjoy sound health in the most flavorful way possible!

Acknowledgments

As *Diabetic Meals in 30 Minutes—or Less!* continues to enjoy popularity after these past 10 years, I must continue to thank the many people with diabetes who have supported my work. Your e-mails and letters have inspired me to continue doing good work. You remind me that it is possible to help people through healthy eating.

I must also thank the American Diabetes Association and all of the editors in the Publications Division for their outstanding guidance and support.

Finally, I owe thanks to my husband Allan, who still eats anything I put in front of him!

INTRODUCTION

HOW THIS BOOK WILL SAVE YOU TIME

Imagine your day as a clock. Do you spend too much of your valuable time on food preparation? Or are you unable to squeeze out any time to prepare nutritious meals without relying on unhealthy and boring prepackaged food? This book will show you how to create wonderful meals without losing precious time for the other things you need to do. This introduction describes some tips that will help you make the best use of this book.

- Preparation times are given for each recipe. This is the time it takes to prepare the ingredients for the recipe, but marinating time and cooking time are not included. Most of these recipes have very short cooking times, however. Marinating is a great technique to use because it adds so much flavor to meats, and you can marinate a meal overnight, thus shortening the actual preparation and cooking time. The goal of this book is to save time, but also to help you prepare interesting food with great flavor.

- To help you improve efficiency in the kitchen, this book outlines dozens of organization tips. You may find, with practice, that your own preparation times may be shorter than those listed here!

- Every effort has been made to assure a quality product. Therefore, the recipes often call for fresh ingredients (especially fruits, vegetables, and herbs) and only include prepackaged food products when their use is necessary and does not affect the recipe's flavor. By practicing the time-saving skills presented here, you will find that using fresh ingredients does not add substantially to the recipe preparation times.

- Reduced-calorie margarine and artificial sweeteners are used very rarely. When reduced-calorie margarine is used, it is to assure the texture of the product. Try to use monounsaturated fats, such as canola or olive oil, instead of reduced-calorie margarine, which can be high in an unhealthy substance called *trans* fats.

- To keep the fats out (or at least down), but keep great flavor in, most of the vegetables are sautéed in small amounts of olive oil. Use a nonstick skillet so the food doesn't burn. If necessary, add a little broth or wine to keep the food from burning (not included in nutrient analyses). Using a nonstick skillet helps save time in cleanup, too.
- Remember, food was meant to be enjoyed and savored! You'll find that these recipes will soon become a valuable part of your healthy, and satisfying, meal plan. *Bon appetit!*

ORGANIZATION 101

Cooking quickly does not mean night after night of the same boring foods. Getting organized from the planning stage through the actual food preparation and cleanup will save you hours of wasted time! Here's how.

Meal Planning

Cooking several days' worth of meals involves planning ahead. Decide before you go to the grocery store what you want to cook, and you'll avoid those pesky repeat trips for a few forgotten items. A well-thought-out plan saves you time and money.

- Start by looking through this book and decide what recipes you would like to prepare for the next week. Plan to make enough food to have leftovers for lunches. You can prepare some of the meat and fish recipes for dinner, then combine the leftovers with salad fixings for a quick lunch. Or, prepare five or six dinners and plan to have leftovers one or two nights a week. This saves you from having to prepare seven different dinners each week.
- Prepare your plan on paper, or, if you are computer savvy, prepare a weekly menu on your computer so you can save and retrieve it whenever you need it. Try to avoid relying on your memory to create a menu plan. You'll be more organized and efficient if you have your plan in writing.

- Prepare your shopping list from your plan. Organize the list like the layout of your grocery store, usually starting with the produce department. Work your way around the perimeter of the store first and then go down the aisles. Most of the food you should be shopping for will be located on the perimeter of the store anyway, because this is where the fresh food is stocked.

- About once a month, shop for staples. You will save lots of time during your weekly trips if your home is already stocked with the bulk of your dry goods. You may want to think a little like a restaurant manager does and always buy a standard quantity of the staples you quickly go through, so you are never caught short. For example, your standard quantity for onions may be one prepackaged bag, because you will probably use onions in many recipes and they keep well in your pantry. Look to see what staples you go through quickly and establish a personal standard quantity for them.

- Try to shop on the same day each week if you can. That way, efficient weekly shopping will become part of your normal routine, rather than several frantic, last-minute affairs.

- Although it is tempting to shop for bargains, think twice about driving to more than three or four stores to find them. The costs of time spent and gas used may not be worth the savings in the bargain you find. Always try to look for the best-quality food you can find.

- As you plan your menus, check to see what you already have in the refrigerator, freezer, and pantry. Many people are surprised to find what they already have on hand. See **What's in the Cupboard: Quick Fixes** for meal ideas that you can prepare from kitchen staples, p. 10.

- When planning a meal, try not to rely on recipes that call for too many pieces of kitchen equipment that you'll have to clean later. Instead, use as few items as possible. For example, if you are preparing casserole-type meals in which everything is mixed together, mix your ingredients right in the casserole dish that you plan to use to bake the meal. That way, cleanup will be much quicker.

- A few times a week, plan on making recipes for one-pot meals. You'll get all of your vegetables, protein, and starch in one pot, making for easy meal planning, short shopping time, and quick cleanup.

- When planning an entire meal, select recipes that don't all require the oven or stove. You may run out of room or waste time waiting for one part of the meal to finish baking before the other part can go in the oven. If you can, cook some of the meal in advance, so you're not in a last-minute panic trying to get all of the food served at the right temperature and at the right time.

- Trying new recipes and using new ingredients is fun and adventurous. But you'll save time relying on and stocking familiar ingredients that you know you'll use time and time again. Going out of your way to purchase an exotic ingredient and not being able to use that ingredient again may not be worth the trouble.

Kitchen Organization

Inefficiency in the kitchen stops many people from preparing delicious, fresh meals. A kitchen that is easy to work in will make cooking more pleasurable and will save you time, too. Here are some ways to get your kitchen organized.

- Take a little time to review all of your kitchen equipment. Just like cleaning out your clothes closet, if an item hasn't been used in years or is damaged, toss it. You won't miss it if you never use it. Make a written list of all of the kitchen equipment you are saving.

- Look carefully at your usual cooking style and how often you need to prepare meals. For example, if you're cooking for one, it might be easier for you to just chop a few vegetables by hand, rather than lugging out that big food processor for a few ingredients.

- Get rid of equipment that is used to make unhealthy food, such as fondue pots and deep-fat fryers. Even if these items are precious wedding gifts, at best they will only collect dust in your cupboard and at worst you'll be making high-fat mistakes with them. Your body will thank you!

- Put items that you use frequently in the same place. Nothing slows down your cooking time more than hunting for an item and finding it in some obscure place. Store seldom-used items in your basement or closet, away from items that you use every day.

- If you have kitchen counter space, place frequently used condiments, grains, and pastas in pretty containers right on or near the counter where you prepare your food. It's quicker to reach for them there than to dig through cabinets. If you do not have spare counter space, but extra kitchen space, consider purchasing a small rolling cart for these frequently used items. You will also be able to quickly tell when you need to replenish your stock!

- Your knives should never be placed in a drawer—this ruins their sharpness. Store them in a wooden block or hang a magnetic strip made for hanging knives (most kitchen shops sell them) on the backsplash of your kitchen wall. Place the knives upright onto the strip for easy access.

What to Buy

These items will make your culinary life more pleasant!

- Buy the best knives you can afford. A well-made carbon steel knife is invaluable, no matter how frequently you cook. Food is much easier to prepare with a high-quality set of knives. You'll need at least an 8- or 10-inch chef's knife for most of your chopping, a paring knife for smaller foods, and a good bread knife.

- Purchase at least one nonstick skillet. They save you time in cleanup and are more healthful to cook with.

- A pasta pot with a steamer/colander insert is a wonderful way to drain pasta without the chore of lifting the pasta to drain in the sink. The steamer insert can also be used to cook vegetables and fish.

- A wok is the most versatile piece of kitchen equipment you can invest in. Besides quick stir-frying, a wok is useful for steaming foods (place a rack inside) and, if it is deep enough, can even be used for making soup. A nonstick wok will save you cleanup time.

- A food processor is useful for big jobs of slicing and shredding. However, make sure you have the room to store one. Be prepared to clean it every time you use it. Consider starting with a smaller version to see how often you really use it. Avoid using a food processor for chopping vegetables with a high water content, such as onions. One second too long and you'll have onion soup!

MEAL PREPARATION

The time you'll save in the kitchen is time you can devote to other healthy pursuits, such as exercising or being with family and friends. Even if you enjoy the time you spend cooking, these tips will add to your culinary efficiency and overall pleasure.

Easy Ways to Prepare Vegetables

Healthy food is often flavored with onion and garlic. These two ingredients can replace much of the flavor that is lost when excess fat and sodium are removed. Here are some easy ways to work with onion, garlic, and the other vegetables that you'll frequently use.

• To chop onions with ease, first slice the onion into two pieces lengthwise, keeping the root end on. Then peel the skin on each half, again keeping the root end on. Make three vertical slices without cutting through the end. Then make several horizontal slices, without cutting through the end. Then turn the onion and proceed to slice downward. You will have uniformly diced onions, and a minimum of onion tears!

To prepare flavorful garlic, chop it by hand rather than using a garlic press. Lay the garlic clove on a working surface and place the flat side of a large knife blade against it. Carefully smack the blade with your fist. This flattens the garlic and makes the skin easy to remove. Make a few cuts with the knife vertically, and then chop.

After you have chopped onions and garlic, you can freeze them for future use. Just spread the chopped vegetables onto a small, nonstick cookie sheet. Spreading them out prevents them from clumping together in a ball when frozen. Cover with plastic wrap and place the sheet in the freezer for 2 hours. When frozen, scrape the onions and garlic into plastic freezer bags. Put about 1/2 to 1 cup at a time in a bag. When recipes call for cooking onions or garlic, just remove your prechopped frozen vegetable from the freezer and begin to cook. Add 2–3 minutes to cooking time. This technique is a real time saver! For fresh salads and cold foods, however, it is best to use fresh onions and garlic.

- Slicing mushrooms is easy with an egg slicer. Just stem the mushrooms and place them in the slicer for even slices.

- Snip herbs right into the pot with a pair of scissors. Use the stems of the herbs, except for tough stems, such as those on rosemary and sage.

- Prepare vegetables one day ahead of time and place them in plastic bags to save time. Try to do this only one day in advance. If you wait longer than that, the vegetables will begin to lose their vitamin content and freshness.

- If you are preparing several recipes together, read through all of them first. If the recipes have similar ingredients that need to be chopped or sliced, do all of your chopping or slicing at the same time.

- When you bring salad greens home, wash them first in a salad spinner to remove any dirt, then wrap the greens with damp paper towels, and place them in a plastic bag. They will stay fresh for an extra day.

Time-Saving Tips

- Always, always read the recipe through at least once before beginning to use it! You might find an ingredient that needs to marinate overnight. Choose another recipe for tonight's dinner and enjoy the marinated meat tomorrow.

- Most marinades and salad dressings can be made in advance. Most of the marinades and dressings in this book will keep in a refrigerated screw-top jar for 1–3 days before you prepare the rest of the recipe.

- Prepare rice, especially long-cooking brown rice, in advance (for tips, see **Tips for Success,** p. 59).

- Learn to dovetail when you cook. It's an efficient way to make use of your time! While a sauce is simmering or a food is marinating, get busy preparing the next step in the recipe or go on to the next dish. You will find out more about how to dovetail in the **Complete Menus** section (p. 139).

- Just like you set aside time to go grocery shopping each week, set aside a window of time to regularly cook each day. We are an appointment-oriented society, so make a "date" with yourself to prepare healthy meals. Make cooking fun by putting on great music to listen to or by sharing the cooking tasks with family members or friends. Have children help, too. Three-year-olds can place cut vegetables in a bag and mix ingredients together. If it's too distracting or unsafe having small children around in the kitchen, plan on cooking when children are otherwise occupied.

- Consider freezing leftovers for later use. Soups, stews, and other casserole dishes freeze well. Line casserole dishes with foil, place the casserole inside, and freeze. Once the food is frozen, lift it out of the dish by its foil edges, wrap with more foil, and return to the freezer. Then wash your dish and store it.

- Make sure your work surface is free of clutter, such as papers, used dishes, and toys. Keep the kitchen ready for food preparation.

- Make sure the lighting in your kitchen is good. Poor lighting will slow down your cooking time. Think about adding some under-cabinet lighting if you do a lot of work on kitchen counters.

BASIC STORAGE TECHNIQUES

Proper storage is as important as food preparation. What a waste of time if the food you prepare is improperly stored and goes bad! First, make sure your refrigerator and freezer are at the proper temperatures: 40°F or less for the refrigerator and 0°F or less for the freezer.

- Leftover chicken broth can be frozen for future use in ice cube trays. When recipes call for broth, just pop out a cube (about 1 Tbsp each).

- Herbs can also be frozen like broth. Just snip the leftover herb into the trays, cover each cube with water, and freeze. When recipes call for an herb in a hot dish, pop out a cube and add it to the dish.

- Eggs should be left in their original cartons and stored in the back of your refrigerator for best freshness.
- Use chicken within 48 hours and fish within 24 hours for best freshness.
- Consider storing flours in the refrigerator or freezer. Whole-grain flours will keep better in the refrigerator or freezer (this prevents them from becoming rancid).

ARE YOU A PACK RAT?

How many of these apply to you?

My dried herbs and spices are more than 1 year old.

My baking powder and baking soda are more than 1 year old.

My dried pastas and grains are more than 1 year old.

My frozen chicken is more than 8 months old.

My frozen fish is more than 6 months old.

My flour is more than 8 months old.

If you answered "yes" to these questions, get out the tissues, wipe your tears, grab a trash bag, and start tossing! To be most efficient in the kitchen—and produce the best-tasting food—don't keep staples past their prime.

- When purchasing dried herbs and spices, buy the smallest quantity available. When storing bottles, place them where you can see them. That way, you can avoid wasting time hunting around in a crowded cupboard. At kitchen shops, buy raised platforms for spices to make them more visible. Some spice racks fit in a kitchen drawer, so you can arrange your spices in rows and find them easily. Lazy susans are sometimes difficult to use, because spices can fall off and bottles can hide behind each other.
- Keep your baking powder and baking soda for no more than 1 year. Longer than that and their leavening power begins to fade.
- Pastas and grains should also be used within 1 year. If your pasta has little white specks on it, it's too old. To keep them fresh, store pastas and grains in tightly sealed glass containers.

- Use frozen chicken within 8 months and fish within 6 months—sooner than that if you can. Frozen meat and fish will never taste quite as good as when they were fresh.
- Flours, like other grains, should be stored in glass containers. Whole-grain flours, such as whole-wheat flour, should always be kept in the refrigerator. If left at room temperature, whole-grain flours will become rancid due to their bran and germ content. You can even store flour in the freezer without affecting its flavor.

QUALITY CLEANUP

All of your efforts to seek out time-saving recipes will be for nothing if it takes you hours to wash 50 different pots and pans. Let's clean up, efficiently!

- Consider using the same dish for mixing and baking.
- Clean as you go!
- If you are preparing pasta and vegetables, place the pasta in the pot first. Add the vegetables 3–4 minutes before cooking time is up. You'll end up with crisp vegetables and only one pot to wash.
- When grilling, coat the rack with oil or nonstick cooking spray. It will be much easier to clean. When cooking puddings or other sticky foods, also coat the saucepan with nonstick cooking spray to prevent sticking and messy cleanup.
- Keep a small toothbrush next to the sink for hard-to-clean nooks and crannies on graters and strainers.

WHAT'S IN THE CUPBOARD: QUICK FIXES

Many cookbooks will give you a list of items to stock in the pantry, but how do you make a meal from them? The next time you think there's nothing to eat at home, look again! Select one of the following 25 ideas and use the staples you already have—a meal is just moments away.

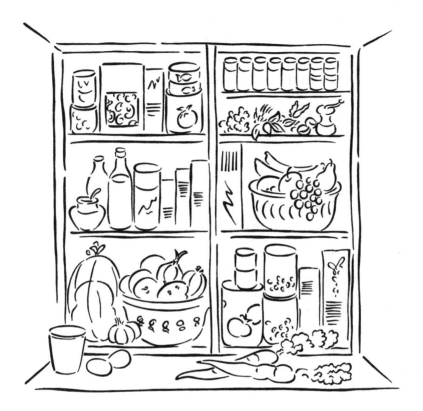

Canned Beans

Beans are not only nutritious, they also add interest to any dish and are easy to prepare. Using canned beans is perfectly acceptable—just rinse them for several minutes under cold running water to get rid of the excess salt. Be sure the beans have no added sugar. You can also freeze cooked beans in a plastic container or freezer bag. Just add cooked frozen beans to a stew or soup and cook it a little longer.

Salsa Salad. Take one 15-oz can drained and rinsed black beans; 2 Tbsp salsa; 1 cup frozen and thawed corn kernels; 1 cup fresh or frozen and thawed carrot slices; 2 Tbsp lime juice; and 1 garlic clove, minced. Combine together and serve. Makes 6 servings.

Salsa Salad: 1 Starch Exchange; 1 Vegetable Exchange; Calories 94; Calories from Fat 3; Total Fat 0 g; Saturated Fat 0 g; Cholesterol 0 mg; Sodium 102 mg; Total Carbohydrate 19 g; Dietary Fiber 5 g; Sugars 3 g; Protein 5 g

Bean Spread. Puree one 15-oz can drained and rinsed kidney or pinto beans with 1 cup low-fat ricotta cheese, 1 tsp ground cumin, 2 tsp chili powder, and 3 Tbsp canned salsa. Puree until smooth. Use as a dip or as a sandwich filling. Makes 16 servings, 2 Tbsp each.

Bean Spread: 1/2 Starch Exchange; Calories 38; Calories from Fat 5; Total Fat 1 g; Saturated Fat 0 g; Cholesterol 6 mg; Sodium 62 mg; Total Carbohydrate 5 g; Dietary Fiber 1 g; Sugars 1 g; Protein 4 g

Zippy Pasta. Take any 15-oz can of beans, drained and rinsed, and combine it with 6 cups cooked pasta. Add 1/2 cup rehydrated dried mushrooms. Add 1/2 cup low-calorie Italian salad dressing and chill. Makes 6 servings.

Zippy Pasta: 3 Starch Exchange; Calories 253; Calories from Fat 27; Total Fat 3 g; Saturated Fat 0 g; Cholesterol 1 mg; Sodium 160 mg; Total Carbohydrate 46 g; Dietary Fiber 6 g; Sugars 4 g; Protein 10 g

Navy Bean Soup. Take one 15-oz can drained and rinsed navy beans and combine with one 28-oz can crushed tomatoes; one 10-oz can low-fat, reduced-sodium chicken broth; 1 cup fresh, sliced, or frozen and thawed zucchini; 1 cup fresh, sliced, or frozen and thawed carrots; 1 tsp each basil and oregano; and 1 cup cooked pasta shells. Heat in a stockpot for 2–3 minutes. Makes 6 servings.

Navy Bean Soup: 1/2 Starch Exchange; 2 Vegetable Exchange; Calories 169; Calories from Fat 10; Total Fat 1 g; Saturated Fat 0 g; Cholesterol 0 mg; Sodium 484 mg; Total Carbohydrate 33 g; Dietary Fiber 7 g; Sugars 9 g; Protein 8 g

Quick Refried Beans. In a skillet over medium-high heat, heat 1 Tbsp olive oil. Add 1 medium chopped onion. Sauté for 5 minutes. Add 2 Tbsp chili powder. Cook for 1 minute. Add one 15-oz can drained and rinsed kidney beans. Mash the beans with a potato masher. Raise the heat to high and cook for 1–2 minutes until beans are a little dry. Makes 6 servings, 1/4 cup each.

Quick Refried Beans: 1 Starch Exchange; 1/2 Fat Exchange; Calories 98; Calories from Fat 26; Total Fat 3 g; Saturated Fat 0 g; Cholesterol 0 mg; Sodium 105 mg; Total Carbohydrate 14 g; Dietary Fiber 4 g; Sugars 3 g; Protein 5 g

Canned Broth

Although it is nice to prepare fresh broth, you won't always have the time. When buying canned broth, look for a low-fat, reduced-sodium variety. Check bouillon cubes for high fat and high sodium content before using them.

Turkey Ball Soup. Heat 3 cups low-fat, reduced-sodium chicken broth. Take 1 lb ground turkey breast meat (your butcher can grind this for you) and combine it with 1 egg, 3 Tbsp dry bread crumbs, 1 Tbsp Worcestershire sauce, and fresh ground pepper and salt to taste. Roll into 1-inch meatballs. Drop into boiling broth and cook until turkey is cooked through, about 10 minutes. Add 1 cup leftover cooked rice or pasta. Cook 1 more minute. Makes 6 servings.

> Turkey Ball Soup: 1/2 Starch Exchange; 3 Very Lean Meat Exchange; Calories 148; Calories from Fat 25; Total Fat 3 g; Saturated Fat 1 g; Cholesterol 86 mg; Sodium 172 mg; Total Carbohydrate 9 g; Dietary Fiber 0 g; Sugars 1 g; Protein 22 g

Clear Asian Soup. Boil 3 cups low-fat, reduced-sodium chicken broth. Add 2 carrots, sliced; 1 celery stalk, sliced; 1 tsp ginger; 1 Tbsp chopped scallions; 2 Tbsp lite soy sauce; 1 Tbsp sherry; and 3 cups cooked pasta. Cook for 10 minutes and enjoy a delicious, quick soup. Makes 6 servings.

> Clear Asian Soup: 1 1/2 Starch Exchange; Calories 112; Calories from Fat 14; Total Fat 2 g; Saturated Fat 0 g; Cholesterol 0 mg; Sodium 280 mg; Total Carbohydrate 21 g; Dietary Fiber 2 g; Sugars 3 g; Protein 5 g

Rice and Pea Soup. Boil 4 cups low-fat, reduced-sodium chicken broth. Add 3 cups cooked leftover brown rice, half of a 10-oz package of frozen peas, and 1 sprig of rosemary. Cook for 5 minutes. Sprinkle with 1 Tbsp grated Parmesan cheese for a comforting soup without fuss. Makes 6 servings.

> Rice and Pea Soup: 2 Starch Exchange; Calories 144; Calories from Fat 24; Total Fat 3 g; Saturated Fat 1 g; Cholesterol 1 mg; Sodium 109 mg; Total Carbohydrate 27 g; Dietary Fiber 3 g; Sugars 2 g; Protein 6 g

Tasty Pasta Soup. Take 3 cups leftover cooked pasta and add it to 4 cups low-fat, reduced-sodium chicken broth. Bring to a boil. Add 1 cup leftover cooked, diced chicken and 1/2 cup canned diced tomatoes. Cook for 5 minutes. Makes 6 servings.

Tasty Pasta Soup: 1 1/2 Starch Exchange; 1 Very Lean Meat Exchange; Calories 162; Calories from Fat 34; Total Fat 4 g; Saturated Fat 1 g; Cholesterol 21 mg; Sodium 92 mg; Total Carbohydrate 22 g; Dietary Fiber 1 g; Sugars 2 g; Protein 12 g

Fast Onion Soup. Heat 1 Tbsp olive oil in a skillet over medium-high heat. Add 3 cups sliced onions. Sauté for 10 minutes, until onions are soft. Add the onions to 6 cups boiling low-fat, reduced-sodium chicken broth. Add 2 Tbsp dry white wine. Grind in pepper. Serve over toasted bread slices in individual bowls. Makes 6 servings.

Fast Onion Soup: 1 Starch Exchange; 1 Vegetable Exchange; 1 Fat Exchange; Calories 149; Calories from Fat 50; Total Fat 6 g; Saturated Fat 1 g; Cholesterol 1 mg; Sodium 244 mg; Total Carbohydrate 2 g; Dietary Fiber 2 g; Sugars 7 g; Protein 6 g

Pasta

Everyone loves pasta. There are so many varieties to choose that you'll never become bored. In addition to the wonderful recipes in this book, here are some fast ideas to combine pasta with other items from your cupboard and refrigerator. Pasta can be prepared and kept in an airtight container for 1 week.

Pasta Pie. To 6 cups cooked spaghetti, add 1 beaten egg white, 1 Tbsp olive oil, 1 Tbsp grated Parmesan cheese, and 2 tsp dried oregano. Combine well. Place in a 9-inch glass pie plate. Bake for 15 minutes, until pasta is slightly browned. Fill the center with 2 cups cooked vegetables. Makes 6 servings.

Pasta Pie: 3 Starch Exchange; Calories 239; Calories from Fat 33; Total Fat 4 g; Saturated Fat 1 g; Cholesterol 1 mg; Sodium 40 mg; Total Carbohydrate 42 g; Dietary Fiber 4 g; Sugars 3 g; Protein 9 g

Artichoke Pasta Salad. Combine 6 cups cooked, cooled, small shell pasta with one 14-oz can water-packed artichoke hearts; 1/2 package frozen and thawed peas; 10 rehydrated, sun-dried tomatoes; and 1/2 cup low-fat salad dressing. Toss well and serve on lettuce. Makes 6 servings.

Artichoke Pasta Salad: 3 Starch Exchange; 1 Vegetable Exchange; Calories 265; Calories from Fat 20; Total Fat 2 g; Saturated Fat 0 g; Cholesterol 0 mg; Sodium 415 mg; Total Carbohydrate 50 g; Dietary Fiber 4 g; Sugars 7 g; Protein 9 g

Sesame Noodles. During the last 3 minutes of cooking 6 cups of fettuccine noodles, add one 10-oz package of frozen mixed vegetables (vegetable mixes with corn, peas, or additional pasta are not included in the nutrient analysis). Drain pasta and vegetables. Add 2 tsp sesame oil, 2 Tbsp toasted sesame seeds, and 1/4 cup sliced scallions. Makes 6 servings.

Sesame Noodles: 3 Starch Exchange; 1/2 Fat Exchange; Calories 261; Calories from Fat 49; Total Fat 5 g; Saturated Fat 1 g; Cholesterol 53 mg; Sodium 25 mg; Total Carbohydrate 44 g; Dietary Fiber 3 g; Sugars 4 g; Protein 9 g

Fast Mediterranean Meal. Add one 15-oz can drained chickpeas (also called garbanzo beans) to 6 cups cooked small elbow macaroni. Drizzle in 2 Tbsp balsamic vinegar and 2 tsp olive oil. Sprinkle with 1 Tbsp grated Parmesan cheese. Serve at room temperature. Makes 6 servings.

Fast Mediterranean Meal: 3 1/2 Starch Exchange; Calories 285; Calories from Fat 35; Total Fat 4 g; Saturated Fat 1 g; Cholesterol 1 mg; Sodium 78 mg; Total Carbohydrate 52 g; Dietary Fiber 4 g; Sugars 4 g; Protein 11 g

Rice

Try these quick ideas to jazz up an ordinary rice dish. To store uncooked rice, keep it in an airtight container in the refrigerator or a cool pantry. Try different kinds of rice for a flavor change. To prepare brown rice, follow the directions on p. 59. Brown rice does take longer to prepare, but you can prepare it ahead of time and freeze it for later use. For these recipes, use cooked, leftover rice you have in the refrigerator.

Viva Mexicana. Sauté 1 medium onion in 1 Tbsp olive oil for 4 minutes. Add in 2 tsp chili powder and 3 cups cooked brown or white rice. Add in one 15-oz can drained kidney beans. Top with canned chilies, if desired. Cook 1 minute. Makes 6 servings.

> Viva Mexicana: 2 1/2 Starch Exchange; Calories 197; Calories from Fat 25; Total Fat 3 g; Saturated Fat 0 g; Cholesterol 0 mg; Sodium 90 mg; Total Carbohydrate 36 g; Dietary Fiber 4 g; Sugars 3 g; Protein 7 g

Down by the Bay. Sauté 2 garlic cloves in 2 tsp olive oil for 1 minute. Add in 2 tsp dried oregano and 3 cups cooked rice. Sauté for 2 minutes. Add in one 10-oz package frozen chopped spinach, thawed and drained well. Add in one 7-oz can baby shrimp. Cook 1 minute. Makes 6 servings.

> Down by the Bay: 1 1/2 Starch Exchange; 1 Very Lean Meat Exchange; Calories 169; Calories from Fat 22; Total Fat 2 g; Saturated Fat 0 g; Cholesterol 57 mg; Sodium 87 mg; Total Carbohydrate 25 g; Dietary Fiber 1 g; Sugars 1 g; Protein 11 g

Fast Fried Rice. In a wok over medium-high heat, heat 2 tsp peanut oil. Add in 2 garlic cloves, minced, and 2 Tbsp sliced scallions. Stir-fry for 30 seconds. Add in 3 cups cooked white or brown rice. Stir-fry for 2 minutes. Add in 1/4 cup lite soy sauce; half of a 10-oz package frozen peas, thawed; and 1 cup bean sprouts. Stir-fry for 2 minutes. Makes 6 servings.

> Fast Fried Rice: 2 Starch Exchange; Calories 145; Calories from Fat 16; Total Fat 2 g; Saturated Fat 0 g; Cholesterol 0 mg; Sodium 425 mg; Total Carbohydrate 28 g; Dietary Fiber 2 g; Sugars 3 g; Protein 4 g

Rice Crust Pizza. Take 3 cups cooked white or brown rice. Add 1 egg, beaten; 2 Tbsp freshly grated Parmesan cheese; and 2 tsp basil. Mix well. Press into a round 12-inch pizza pan. Spread evenly. Bake in a 350°F preheated oven for 10 minutes. Top with 1 cup shredded, fat-free mozzarella cheese, 1 cup reduced-fat pizza sauce, 1 cup mushrooms, and 1 cup sliced red or green pepper. Return to the oven and bake until cheese melts. Makes 6 servings.

Rice Crust Pizza: 1 1/2 Starch Exchange; 1 Vegetable Exchange; 1 Lean Meat Exchange; Calories 184; Calories from Fat 22; Total Fat 2 g; Saturated Fat 0.8 g; Cholesterol 40 mg; Sodium 427 mg; Total Carbohydrate 28 g; Dietary Fiber 2 g; Sugars 4 g; Protein 10 g

Canned Fish

In a pinch, canned fish will work well. Buy canned tuna and salmon that is packed in water. Canned salmon is a particularly good source of calcium, with its edible soft bones. For best results, buy solid white tuna and pink salmon.

Tuna Pâté. In a blender, puree 1 cup 1% cottage cheese, 2 Tbsp scallions, 1 tsp minced parsley, 2 tsp minced dill, and 2 tsp lite soy sauce. Add one 7-oz can drained tuna. Blend again until smooth. Spread the tuna pâté on sandwiches or serve from a crock with crackers. Makes 6 servings.

Tuna Pâté: 2 Very Lean Meat Exchange; Calories 61; Calories from Fat 5; Total Fat 1 g; Saturated Fat 0 g; Cholesterol 10 mg; Sodium 315 mg; Total Carbohydrate 1 g; Dietary Fiber 0 g; Sugars 1 g; Protein 12 g

Salmon Niçoise. Toss together one 16-oz can pink salmon; one 10-oz package frozen green beans, thawed and drained; one 14-oz can artichoke hearts, drained; 1 red pepper, diced; and 1/2 cup low-calorie Italian salad dressing. Toss well and serve. Makes 6 servings.

Salmon Niçoise: 2 Vegetable Exchange; 2 Lean Meat Exchange; Calories 161; Calories from Fat 57; Total Fat 6 g; Saturated Fat 1 g; Cholesterol 31 mg; Sodium 648 mg; Total Carbohydrate 8 g; Dietary Fiber 3 g; Sugars 4 g; Protein 18 g

Tonnato Sauce. In a skillet over medium-high heat, heat 2 tsp olive oil. Add 1 medium onion, diced. Sauté for 4 minutes. Add 2 cups crushed tomatoes, 2 Tbsp dry red wine, and 2 tsp dried oregano. Bring to a boil. Lower the heat and simmer for 10 minutes. Add one

7-oz can tuna, drained. Add in 1 Tbsp capers. Serve sauce over cooked pasta (not included in nutrient analysis). Makes 6 servings.

> Tonnato Sauce: 2 Vegetable Exchange; 1 Very Lean Meat Exchange; Calories 90; Calories from Fat 17; Total Fat 2 g; Saturated Fat 0 g; Cholesterol 8 mg; Sodium 321 mg; Total Carbohydrate 9 g; Dietary Fiber 2 g; Sugars 5 g; Protein 9 g

Couscous Tuna Salad.

Toss one 7-oz can tuna, drained, with 2 cups rehydrated couscous (start out with 1 cup dry couscous, pour 2 cups boiling water over couscous, and let stand for 5 minutes, until water is absorbed); 1/2 cup frozen corn, thawed and drained; 2 Tbsp minced cilantro; 2 Tbsp red wine vinegar; and 1 Tbsp olive oil. Grind in fresh pepper and serve at room temperature. Makes 6 servings.

> Couscous Tuna Salad: 2 Starch Exchange; 1 Very Lean Meat Exchange; Calories 179; Calories from Fat 24; Total Fat 3 g; Saturated Fat 0 g; Cholesterol 8 mg; Sodium 98 mg; Total Carbohydrate 27 g; Dietary Fiber 2 g; Sugars 1 g; Protein 11 g

Quick Salmon Burgers.

Combine one 7-oz can salmon, drained, with 1 egg, beaten; 2 Tbsp Dijon mustard; 3 Tbsp dry bread crumbs; and 2 tsp Tabasco® sauce. Form into patties and place in a heated nonstick skillet. Cook for 5–6 minutes on each side until browned. Makes 6 servings.

> Quick Salmon Burgers: 3 Very Lean Meat Exchange; 1/2 Fat Exchange; Calories 137; Calories from Fat 48; Total Fat 5 g; Saturated Fat 1 g; Cholesterol 65 mg; Sodium 482 mg; Total Carbohydrate 3 g; Dietary Fiber 0 g; Sugars 1 g; Protein 18 g

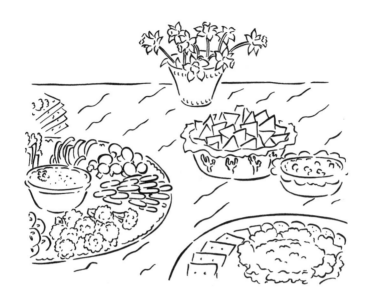

APPEALING APPETIZERS

Traditionally, appetizers are like fat magnets: mini-quiches, wrapped sausages, and sour cream dips all spell disaster for a healthy meal plan!

Fortunately, you can make appetizers that taste good, display attractively, and still provide basic good nutrition. All of the recipes in this chapter can be made in advance, so you can concentrate on your guests when they arrive. If you're not feeling like hosting a party, enjoy them as great snacks instead.

For dipping into the spreads, try all kinds of vegetables, toasted pita wedges, reduced-fat baked tortilla chips, reduced-fat crackers, or mini rice cakes. Try serving the dips in hollowed-out cabbages, zucchini, or yellow squash; colorful pepper cups; a crusty, hollowed-out, round loaf of bread; or a decorative crock.

Host a healthy appetizer party with these easy and delicious recipes!

SPICY HUMMUS

RED PEPPER HUMMUS

BLACK BEAN HUMMUS

SUN-DRIED TOMATO AND BASIL DIP

SPINACH DIP

WHITE BEAN PÂTÉ

SESAME BASIL CHICKEN TIDBITS

FRESH TOMATO BRUSCHETTA

SPICED SCALLOPS

ORIENTAL GINGER PORK

Spicy Hummus

Total Servings: 12
Serving Size: 2 Tbsp

Preparation time: 5 minutes

Everyone likes the Middle Eastern dip called hummus!
Made with garbanzo beans (also called chickpeas), hummus is
high in fiber and protein. Unfortunately, commercially prepared
hummus can be very high in fat, due to the addition of too much
sesame tahini (sesame butter) and oil. Here's a lighter version of
the traditional dip that you can make yourself.

1   15-oz can chickpeas, drained and
       rinsed (reserve 1 Tbsp liquid)
1   Tbsp sesame tahini
3   garlic cloves, minced
1   Tbsp lemon juice
1   tsp olive oil
1   tsp cumin
1   tsp coriander
1/2 tsp cayenne pepper
     Fresh ground white pepper
2   tsp minced parsley

Exchanges	
1/2 Starch	
Calories	48
Calories from Fat	15
Total Fat	2 g
Saturated Fat	0 g
Cholesterol	0 mg
Sodium	34 mg
Total Carbohydrate	7 g
Dietary Fiber	1 g
Sugars	1 g
Protein	2 g

Combine all ingredients in a blender or food processor. Use 1 Tbsp of
reserved bean juice to moisten, if necessary. Process until smooth.

Red Pepper Hummus

Total Servings: 12
Serving Size: 2 Tbsp

This recipe contains sesame tahini, but considerably less than store-bought hummus.

1/2 cup canned chickpeas, drained
2 roasted red peppers (purchase roasted red peppers in a jar from the condiment aisle in your grocery store)
1 Tbsp sesame tahini
2 Tbsp plain reduced-fat yogurt
2 garlic cloves, minced
1 Tbsp minced onion
Dash cayenne pepper
Fresh ground pepper to taste

Exchanges	
1 Vegetable	
Calories	28
Calories from Fat	13
Total Fat	1 g
Saturated Fat	0 g
Cholesterol	0 mg
Sodium	69 mg
Total Carbohydrate	3 g
Dietary Fiber	1 g
Sugars	2 g
Protein	1 g

Combine the first three ingredients in a blender or food processor until smooth. Add the remaining ingredients and process until smooth.

Black Bean Hummus

Total Servings: 12
Serving Size: 2 Tbsp

Preparation time: 8 minutes

Serve this dip with fat-free tortilla chips, pita bread wedges, or raw vegetables.

1 15-oz can black beans, drained
1 Tbsp sesame tahini
1 Tbsp reduced-fat sour cream
4 garlic cloves, minced
1 Tbsp minced tomato
1 Tbsp lime juice
1 tsp cumin
   Fresh ground pepper to taste

Exchanges	
1/2 Starch	
Calories	43
Calories from Fat	8
Total Fat	1 g
Saturated Fat	0 g
Cholesterol	0 mg
Sodium	45 mg
Total Carbohydrate	7 g
Dietary Fiber	2 g
Sugars	1 g
Protein	2 g

Combine all ingredients in a blender or food processor. Process until smooth.

Sun-Dried Tomato and Basil Dip

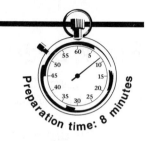

Total Servings: 12
Serving Size: 2 Tbsp

This creamy dip can also be used as a salad dressing. Just thin out the mixture with some nonfat milk or reduced-fat buttermilk and mix until smooth and creamy.

1 cup reduced-fat ricotta cheese
4 sun-dried tomatoes, rehydrated and finely minced (Avoid using the sun-dried tomatoes in oil. It is very difficult to remove the high-fat oil from the tomatoes.)
2 garlic cloves, finely minced
1 tsp finely minced chives
1 Tbsp finely minced basil
1 tsp olive oil

Exchanges	
1 Vegetable	
Calories	33
Calories from Fat	10
Total Fat	1 g
Saturated Fat	1 g
Cholesterol	8 mg
Sodium	104 mg
Total Carbohydrate	3 g
Dietary Fiber	0 g
Sugars	1 g
Protein	4 g

Combine all ingredients by hand in a small bowl. Refrigerate until serving time or about 2 hours. This dip is very good served with crackers or raw vegetables.

Spinach Dip

Total Servings: 12
Serving Size: 2 Tbsp

Preparation time: 7 minutes

If you let the spinach defrost in the refrigerator, you can avoid spending time cooking it. You can also use this dip to top broiled salmon steaks.

1   10-oz package frozen chopped
    spinach or broccoli, thawed
2   Tbsp red wine vinegar
3   garlic cloves, minced
1   Tbsp fresh minced mint
1   cup reduced-fat sour cream
    Fresh ground pepper to taste

Exchanges	
1 Vegetable	
Calories	26
Calories from Fat	14
Total Fat	2 g
Saturated Fat	1 g
Cholesterol	7 mg
Sodium	24 mg
Total Carbohydrate	2 g
Dietary Fiber	1 g
Sugars	1 g
Protein	1 g

Drain the defrosted spinach and press out all of the water until the spinach is very dry. Combine all ingredients by hand. Refrigerate for 2 hours. Serve inside a hollowed-out, round loaf of bread and surround with crackers, breadsticks, vegetables, or pita wedges.

White Bean Pâté

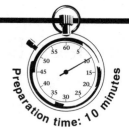

Total Servings: 12
Serving Size: 2 Tbsp

This spread resembles the wonderfully aromatic French boursin cheese, but contains much less fat.

1/2 cup minced scallions
3 garlic cloves, minced
1 15-oz can white beans (navy or cannellini)
2 tsp prepared Dijon mustard
1 Tbsp fresh lemon juice
1 tsp olive oil
2 Tbsp minced parsley
1 Tbsp minced basil
1 tsp minced thyme leaves
1 tsp minced dill
1 tsp minced tarragon
1/4 tsp nutmeg
Fresh ground pepper and salt to taste

Exchange
1/2 Starch
Calories 49
Calories from Fat 5
Total Fat .... 1 g
Saturated Fat .... 0 g
Cholesterol .... 0 mg
Sodium .... 165 mg
Total Carbohydrate . 9 g
Dietary Fiber .... 2 g
Sugars .... 1 g
Protein .... 3 g

Combine all ingredients in a blender or food processor. Process until smooth. Serve with crackers or pita bread.

Sesame Basil Chicken Tidbits

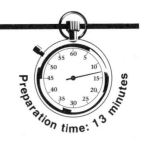

Preparation time: 13 minutes

Total Servings: 6
Serving Size: 2 oz

These tender little chicken bites can be made ahead of time and reheated at the last moment. Since the chicken has been marinated, it will not lose its moistness.

Chicken
3/4 lb boneless, skinless chicken breasts

Marinade
3 Tbsp lite soy sauce
2 tsp sesame oil
2 Tbsp dry sherry
2 Tbsp fresh orange juice
2 Tbsp minced fresh basil
1 Tbsp toasted sesame seeds
2 dried red chilies

Red leaf lettuce to line platter

Exchanges	
2 Very Lean Meat	
Calories	79
Calories from Fat	20
Total Fat	2 g
Saturated Fat	1 g
Cholesterol	34 mg
Sodium	131 mg
Total Carbohydrate	1 g
Dietary Fiber	0 g
Sugars	1 g
Protein	13 g

1. Cut the chicken breasts into 2-inch cubes.

2. Combine all of the marinade ingredients and mix well. Add the cubed chicken and marinate in the refrigerator for at least 2 hours.

3. Remove the chicken cubes from the marinade and place on a broiler rack. Broil 2–3 minutes per side, until chicken is cooked throughout.

4. Serve on a lettuce-lined platter with fancy frill toothpicks.

Fresh Tomato Bruschetta

Total Servings: 6
Serving Size: 1 oz

Preparation time: 10 minutes

This is the simplest of appetizers, yet elegant enough for any party.

Bread

1   6-oz loaf Italian or French bread
1   Tbsp olive oil

Topping

2   plum tomatoes, minced (or 1 salad tomato)
3   garlic cloves, minced
2   tsp minced basil
1   tsp minced thyme
2   tsp olive oil

Exchanges	
1 Starch	
1 Fat	
Calories	118
Calories from Fat	22
Total Fat	4 g
Saturated Fat	0 g
Cholesterol	0 mg
Sodium	156 mg
Total Carbohydrate	16 g
Dietary Fiber	2 g
Sugars	2 g
Protein	2 g

1   Preheat the oven to 350°F. Cut the bread into 6 even slices. Brush each slice with olive oil and place onto a cookie sheet.

2. To prepare the topping, combine all ingredients.

3. Place the bread in the oven and toast for 1–2 minutes.

4. Remove the bread from the oven and spread a teaspoon of topping over each slice. Serve immediately.

Spiced Scallops

Total Servings: 6
Serving Size: about 2 oz

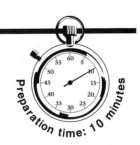

Zippy spices jazz up mild bay scallops.

Spice mixture
- 2 Tbsp fresh lemon juice
- 1 medium onion, chopped
- 3 garlic cloves, minced
- 1/4 cup minced parsley
- 3 tsp cumin
- 1 tsp cayenne pepper
- 1 tsp coriander
- Fresh ground pepper to taste
- Tabasco® sauce to taste

Scallops
- 3/4 lb bay scallops

Exchanges	
1 Very Lean Meat	
Calories	50
Calories from Fat	4
Total Fat	0 g
Saturated Fat	0 g
Cholesterol	18 mg
Sodium	92 mg
Total Carbohydrate	2 g
Dietary Fiber	0 g
Sugars	1 g
Protein	9 g

1. Combine all ingredients for spice mixture. Toss the scallops in the mixture. Let them marinate for 20 minutes.

2. In a steamer over boiling water, steam the scallops for about 2 minutes. Remove from heat.

3. Place the scallops on a plate and spear with toothpicks. Serve immediately.

Oriental Ginger Pork

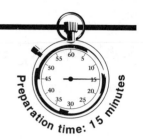

Preparation time: 15 minutes

Total Servings: 6
Serving Size: 2 oz with 1 Tbsp sauce

Keep a good supply of napkins ready for this fun-to-eat appetizer!

Pork

 1 lb lean pork tenderloin, trimmed and ground (your butcher can do this for you)
 2 garlic cloves, minced
 1 tsp ground ginger
 1 tsp lite soy sauce

Sauce

 1/4 cup rice vinegar
 1/2 cup lite soy sauce
 1/4 cup tomato paste
 2 Tbsp honey
 1 Tbsp Tabasco® sauce

Exchange	
1/2 Starch	
2 Very Lean Meat	
Calories	107
Calories from Fat	25
Total Fat	3 g
Saturated Fat	1 g
Cholesterol	44 mg
Sodium	341 mg
Total Carbohydrate	4 g
Dietary Fiber	0 g
Sugars	3 g
Protein	16 g

1. Preheat the oven to 350°F. Combine the pork with the garlic, ginger, and soy sauce. Form into 2-inch meatballs.

2. Combine all sauce ingredients and set aside.

3. Place meatballs in a baking dish and bake for 20 minutes. Add the sauce and bake for 10 more minutes. Serve meatballs speared with toothpicks.

Diabetic Meals in 30 Minutes—Or Less!

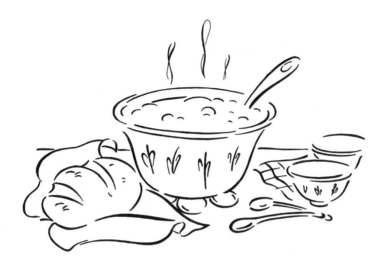

Soup's On!

Serving a hearty soup is a great way to get a meal on the table in no time flat. Just add cooked or raw vegetables and some crusty bread to complete the meal! All of the following soups can be frozen for future use. You can freeze soup in heavy-duty plastic zip-top freezer bags or 1-quart containers. To reheat the soup, defrost it in the microwave first on the defrost setting and then continue to heat until the soup is at the desired temperature.

All of these soups make use of canned low-fat, reduced-sodium broths. When you have more time, consider making your own broth. When you shop for canned broth, look for a brand that has a clear broth with very little fat resting on the top when you open it. Any leftover broth can be saved for future use. Just pour it into ice cube trays and freeze. When recipes call for broth, just pop out a cube (about 1 Tbsp each).

Grab a bowl and savor these fresh homemade soups!

ROASTED RED PEPPER SOUP

CREAMY CORN CHOWDER

SPEEDY BLACK BEAN SOUP

QUICK CHILI

55 60 5

TUSCAN BEAN SOUP

50   10

CREAMY PUMPKIN SOUP

45   15

40   20

GOLDEN BUTTERNUT SQUASH SOUP

35 25

30

HOT AND SOUR SOUP

COD AND SHRIMP SOUP

Roasted Red Pepper Soup

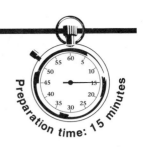

Preparation time: 15 minutes

Total Servings: 6
Serving Size: 1 cup

Serve this rosy red soup any time of the year.

Soup

2	Tbsp olive oil
1	medium onion, chopped
4	garlic cloves, minced
3	roasted red peppers or 1 7-oz jar (roasted red peppers in a jar are in the grocery store condiment aisle)
3	cups low-fat, reduced-sodium chicken broth
1/2	cup tomato juice
	Fresh ground pepper to taste

Garnish

Paper-thin lemon slices
Parsley sprigs
Fresh ground pepper to taste

Exchanges	
1/2 Starch	
1 Fat	
Calories	80
Calories from Fat	54
Total Fat	6 g
Saturated Fat	1 g
Cholesterol	0 mg
Sodium	300 mg
Total Carbohydrate	7 g
Dietary Fiber	1 g
Sugars	6 g
Protein	3 g

1. In a small skillet over medium-high heat, heat the oil. Add the onion and garlic and sauté for 5 minutes. Do not let garlic turn brown. Remove from heat.

2. In a blender or food processor, place the garlic onion mixture and the roasted red peppers. Puree until smooth.

3. In a stockpot over high heat, bring the broth to a boil. Lower the heat to medium and add the roasted pepper puree. Stir until smooth. Add the tomato juice and simmer for 10 minutes. Add the pepper.

4. To serve, pour soup into soup bowls. Place 2 slices of lemon per bowl in the center of the bowl. Top with a parsley sprig. Grind more black pepper on top. Serve immediately.

Creamy Corn Chowder

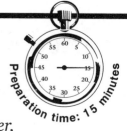

Total Servings: 6
Serving Size: 1 cup

This chowder is rich and satisfying. In the summer, use fresh corn scraped right off the cob.

Chowder

- 1 tsp olive oil
- 1 medium onion, chopped
- 1 medium potato, peeled and diced
- 1 cup low-fat, reduced-sodium chicken broth
- 2 cups corn kernels
- 2 cups evaporated nonfat milk
- 2 Tbsp cornstarch or arrowroot
- 4 Tbsp cold water
  Fresh ground pepper to taste
- 1 tsp liquid smoke (optional)

Garnish

- 2 Tbsp minced parsley

Exchanges	
2 Starch	
Calories	156
Calories from Fat	13
Total Fat	1 g
Saturated Fat	0 g
Cholesterol	3 mg
Sodium	121 mg
Total Carbohydrate	29 g
Dietary Fiber	2 g
Sugars	10 g
Protein	9 g

1. In a nonstick stockpot, heat the oil. Add the onion and sauté for 5 minutes. Add the diced potato and 1/2 cup of the broth. Cook for 10 minutes, until potato is soft.

2. Add the corn, milk, and remaining broth and simmer over medium heat for 15 minutes.

3. Combine the cornstarch and water. Add to the soup and cook over low heat until soup is thickened. Add liquid smoke, if desired. Garnish with parsley.

Speedy Black Bean Soup

Total Servings: 6
Serving Size: 1 cup

Preparation time: 15 minutes

There are many versions of Black Bean Soup available, but this one is probably the fastest around. No vegetables are included, except onion, so if you want to include more vegetables, the soup will take a little longer to cook.

Soup

- 1 tsp olive oil
- 1 small onion, minced
- 2 15-oz cans black beans, 1 can drained
- 1 1/2 cups low-fat, reduced-sodium chicken broth
- 1/2 cup dry red wine
- Fresh ground pepper to taste
- 1 tsp cayenne pepper

Garnish

- 6 Tbsp reduced-fat sour cream
- Cilantro or parsley sprigs

Exchanges	
1 1/2 Starch	
1 Very Lean Meat	
Calories	168
Calories from Fat	27
Total Fat	3 g
Saturated Fat	1 g
Cholesterol	5 mg
Sodium	394 mg
Total Carbohydrate	26 g
Dietary Fiber	8 g
Sugars	4 g
Protein	10 g

1. In a stockpot over medium-high heat, heat the oil. Add the onion and sauté for 5 minutes.

2. Add the drained can of beans and chicken broth. Simmer for 5 minutes.

3. Puree the other can of beans with the bean liquid in a blender or food processor. Add to the soup. Add the red wine, ground pepper, and cayenne pepper and simmer for 10 minutes. Garnish with sour cream and parsley or cilantro sprigs.

Quick Chili

Total Servings: 6
Serving Size: 1 cup

*True chili is actually prepared without beans. This
soup simmers just long enough for the flavors to blend.*

2 tsp olive oil	
1 medium onion, chopped	
1 small red pepper, chopped	
4 cloves garlic, minced	
1 lb lean pork tenderloin, trimmed and ground (your butcher can do this for you)	
3 Tbsp ground chili powder	
1 tsp cinnamon	
1/2 tsp allspice	
2 cups canned tomatoes, coarsely chopped, undrained	
2 cups reduced-sodium beef broth	
1 Tbsp red wine	
1 Tbsp Worcestershire sauce	
Fresh ground pepper to taste	

Exchanges
1/2 Starch
2 Lean Meat

Calories 160
Calories from Fat 53
Total Fat .... 6 g
Saturated Fat .... 1 g
Cholesterol .... 44 mg
Sodium .... 262 mg
Total Carbohydrate 11 g
Dietary Fiber .... 3 g
Sugars .... 5 g
Protein .... 18 g

1. In a stockpot over medium-high heat, heat the oil. Add the onion and pepper and sauté for 5 minutes. Add the garlic and sauté for 2 minutes. Add the pork and sauté for 5 minutes.

2. Add the remaining ingredients and simmer over medium-low heat for 20 minutes.

Diabetic Meals in 30 Minutes—Or Less!

Tuscan Bean Soup

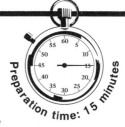

Preparation time: 15 minutes

Total Servings: 6
Serving Size: 1 cup

This hearty soup, plus bread and salad, is all you need for a filling meal.

1 Tbsp olive oil
1 medium onion, minced
2 garlic cloves, minced
1 medium red pepper, chopped
3 cups low-fat, reduced-sodium chicken broth
1 cup coarsely chopped canned tomatoes
1 1/2 cups canned red kidney beans, cannellini beans, or navy beans, drained
2 tsp chopped fresh thyme
1/2 cup chopped spinach or escarole
1 cup cooked small pasta shells
Fresh ground pepper to taste

Exchanges	
2 Starch	
1/2 Fat	
Calories	184
Calories from Fat	56
Total Fat	6 g
Saturated Fat	1 g
Cholesterol	0 mg
Sodium	212 mg
Total Carbohydrate	27 g
Dietary Fiber	4 g
Sugars	5 g
Protein	8 g

1. In a stockpot over medium-high heat, heat the oil. Add the onion and garlic and sauté for 5 minutes. Add the pepper and sauté for 3 more minutes.

2. Add the broth, tomatoes, and beans. Bring to a boil. Simmer over low heat for 20 minutes.

3. Add the thyme, spinach or escarole, and cooked pasta. Simmer for 5 more minutes. Grind in pepper to taste and serve.

Creamy Pumpkin Soup

Total Servings: 6
Serving Size: 1 cup

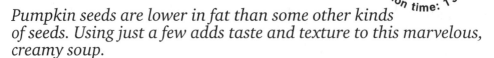

Pumpkin seeds are lower in fat than some other kinds of seeds. Using just a few adds taste and texture to this marvelous, creamy soup.

1/4 cup pumpkin seeds	
2 tsp canola oil	
1 medium onion, chopped	
1 1/2 cups canned pumpkin	
3 1/2 cups low-fat, reduced-sodium chicken broth	
1 cup evaporated nonfat milk	
2 Tbsp dry sherry	
1 tsp cinnamon	
Fresh ground pepper to taste	

Exchanges

1 Starch
1 1/2 Fat

Calories	142
Calories from Fat	64
Total Fat	7 g
Saturated Fat	1 g
Cholesterol	2 mg
Sodium	115 mg
Total Carbohydrate	14 g
Dietary Fiber	3 g
Sugars	8 g
Protein	9 g

1. Preheat the oven to 400°F. Spread the pumpkin seeds on a small cookie sheet. Drizzle 1 tsp of the canola oil on the seeds and toast the seeds for 5 minutes. Remove from the oven.

2. In a stockpot, heat the remaining oil. Add the onion and sauté for 5 minutes. Add the pumpkin and broth and bring to a boil. Simmer for 20 minutes. Add the milk, sherry, and cinnamon. Simmer for 5 minutes.

3. To serve, place soup in bowls and top with pumpkin seeds. Grind pepper over each serving.

Golden Butternut Squash Soup

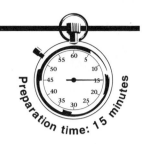

Preparation time: 15 minutes

Total Servings: 6
Serving Size: 1 cup

Butternut squash is a great source of vitamin A. If you use frozen butternut squash, you will save considerable cooking time. If you prefer fresh squash or if you have more time, use 1 1/2 lb cubed raw butternut squash and cook the soup for 45 minutes.

1	tsp canola oil
1	small onion, minced
1	carrot, peeled and diced
2	10-oz packages butternut squash, thawed
1	cup low-fat, reduced-sodium chicken broth
1 1/2	cups evaporated nonfat milk
1	tsp nutmeg
	Fresh ground pepper to taste

Exchanges
1 Starch
1 Vegetable

Calories	110
Calories from Fat	13
Total Fat	1 g
Saturated Fat	0 g
Cholesterol	2 mg
Sodium	107 mg
Total Carbohydrate	20 g
Dietary Fiber	3 g
Sugars	9 g
Protein	7 g

1. In a stockpot over medium-high heat, heat the oil. Add the onion and sauté for 3 minutes. Add the carrot and sauté for 3 more minutes. Add the butternut squash and broth and bring to a boil.

2. Add the milk and simmer on low heat for 20 minutes.

3. Add the nutmeg. In batches, puree the soup in a blender until smooth. Add pepper to taste. Serve immediately.

Hot and Sour Soup

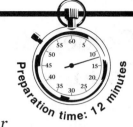

Total Servings: 6
Serving Size: 1 cup

The traditional great taste, but less fat and fewer calories!

4 cups low-fat, reduced-sodium chicken broth
4 Tbsp white vinegar
2 Tbsp lite soy sauce
1 Tbsp crushed red pepper
2 tsp sesame oil
1 cup sliced mushrooms
1 cup thinly sliced carrot
2 tsp cornstarch or arrowroot
4 tsp water

Exchanges	
1/2 Starch	
1/2 Fat	
Calories	50
Calories from Fat	28
Total Fat	3 g
Saturated Fat	1 g
Cholesterol	0 mg
Sodium	288 mg
Total Carbohydrate	6 g
Dietary Fiber	1 g
Sugars	3 g
Protein	3 g

1. In a stockpot, combine the broth, vinegar, soy sauce, crushed red pepper, and sesame oil. Bring to a boil, then simmer for 10 minutes.

2. Add the mushrooms and carrots and simmer for 10 more minutes.

3. Combine the cornstarch or arrowroot with the water. Add it to the soup and continue to cook for 5 minutes, until thickened.

Diabetic Meals in 30 Minutes—Or Less!

Cod and Shrimp Soup

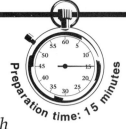

Total Servings: 6
Serving Size: 1 cup with 3 oz seafood

Use this soup as a first course before pasta or with fresh bread and salad for a nutritious meal.

2	tsp olive oil
1	medium onion, minced
3	garlic cloves, minced
1	small red pepper, diced
2	cups canned tomatoes, coarsely chopped, undrained
1	cup sliced okra
1 1/2	cups low-fat, reduced-sodium chicken broth
1	tsp chili powder
1	tsp celery seed
2	tsp paprika
2	Tbsp tomato paste
3/4	lb cod fillets, cubed
2/3	lb shelled and deveined medium shrimp

Exchanges	
1 Starch	
3 Very Lean Meat	
Calories	166
Calories from Fat	34
Total Fat	4 g
Saturated Fat	1 g
Cholesterol	98 mg
Sodium	268 mg
Total Carbohydrate	12 g
Dietary Fiber	3 g
Sugars	6 g
Protein	23 g

1. In a stockpot, heat the oil. Add the onion and garlic and sauté for 3 minutes. Add the red pepper and sauté for 3 more minutes.

2. Add all of the remaining ingredients except the cod and shrimp. Simmer over low heat for 20 minutes.

3. Add the cod and shrimp and cover. Cook for 5 more minutes. Serve immediately.

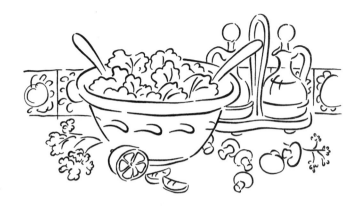

Super Salads

Today a salad means more than just a wedge of iceberg lettuce and Thousand Island dressing! By being creative with different kinds of vegetables, you can turn a humdrum salad into a culinary feast.

Including a fresh salad every day in your meal plan increases your fiber intake. Always try to include dark greens first, such as spinach and romaine lettuce, when choosing salad ingredients.

The culprit that turns relatively healthy salads into diet disasters is the high fat content in most dressings. Instead, enliven the flavor of your salads with interesting vinegars and fresh herbs. The traditional ratio of oil to vinegar is two to one. Reverse that proportion to make an equally delicious, but much lower-fat, salad dressing. Feel free to experiment: try using only vinegar and lots of herbs. You may be surprised to find you don't miss the oil at all!

Dressings should not overpower a salad. Instead, just use a fine mist or splash of dressing to wake up greens. If you find you need more dressing to coat your salad, increase the proportion of nonfat ingredients only, such as the juices and vinegars.

ARUGULA AND WATERCRESS SALAD

WALNUT-FLAVORED ARTICHOKE AND GRAPEFRUIT SALAD

SPINACH ORANGE SALAD

FRESH BEET AND CARROT SALAD

BROCCOLI SALAD

HEALTHY COLESLAW

LOW-FAT DIJON POTATO SALAD

CORIANDER CARROT SALAD

ITALIAN BEAN SALAD

FRESH SNOW PEA AND TRI-COLORED PEPPER SALAD

SLICED TOMATOES WITH ITALIAN PARSLEY DRESSING

Arugula and Watercress Salad

Preparation time: 8 minutes

Total Servings: 6
Serving Size: 1 cup

A great-tasting salad with a bite!

Dressing
    2 Tbsp olive oil
    3 Tbsp sherry vinegar
    1 Tbsp Dijon mustard
    1 Tbsp orange juice
    2 tsp grated orange peel
       Fresh ground pepper and salt to taste

Salad
    4 cups arugula, washed and torn
    2 cups watercress, washed and torn
    1 red onion, sliced into thin rings
 1/2 cup halved cherry tomatoes

Garnish
    2 Tbsp toasted sesame seeds

Exchanges	
1 Vegetable	
1 Fat	
Calories	80
Calories from Fat	56
Total Fat	6 g
Saturated Fat	1 g
Cholesterol	0 mg
Sodium	66 mg
Total Carbohydrate	5 g
Dietary Fiber	1 g
Sugars	3 g
Protein	2 g

1. Combine all dressing ingredients in a small bowl. Whisk until blended.

2. In a salad bowl, toss all ingredients for the salad. Add dressing and toss well.

3. Top each individual salad plate with toasted sesame seeds.

Walnut-Flavored Artichoke and Grapefruit Salad

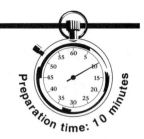

Total Servings: 6
Serving Size: 1 cup

The delicate, yet robust, flavor of walnut oil gives this salad a gourmet touch.

2 Tbsp walnut oil
3 Tbsp white wine vinegar
1 Tbsp minced parsley
1 Tbsp minced scallions
1 15-oz can artichoke hearts, drained
4 cups combined romaine lettuce leaves and endive leaves, washed and torn
1 large pink grapefruit, separated into sections

Exchanges	
1/2 Fruit	
1 Vegetable	
1 Fat	
Calories	82
Calories from Fat	44
Total Fat	5 g
Saturated Fat	0 g
Cholesterol	0 mg
Sodium	122 mg
Total Carbohydrate	9 g
Dietary Fiber	3 g
Sugars	5 g
Protein	2 g

1. Combine the walnut oil, vinegar, parsley, and scallions in a blender. Process 15 seconds. Toss artichoke hearts into the dressing and refrigerate while you prepare the lettuce and grapefruit.

2. Place the lettuce leaves and endive on individual plates or in a large salad bowl. Place the grapefruit sections in a star pattern over the lettuce. Pile the marinated artichokes on top.

Diabetic Meals in 30 Minutes—Or Less!

Spinach Orange Salad

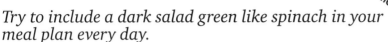

Total Servings: 6
Serving Size: 1 cup

Try to include a dark salad green like spinach in your meal plan every day.

Dressing

- 2 Tbsp canola oil
- 3 Tbsp orange juice
- 1 Tbsp lemon juice
- 1 tsp grated orange peel
  Fresh ground pepper and salt to taste

Salad

- 5 cups torn fresh spinach leaves, washed and dried
- 1/2 cup mandarin oranges, packed in their own juice, drained
- 1/2 cup thinly sliced dried apricots
- 1 small red onion, thinly sliced
- 1 Tbsp toasted pine nuts

Exchanges	
1/2 Fruit	
1 Vegetable	
1 Fat	
Calories	105
Calories from Fat	52
Total Fat	6 g
Saturated Fat	1 g
Cholesterol	0 mg
Sodium	63 mg
Total Carbohydrate	13 g
Dietary Fiber	3 g
Sugars	8 g
Protein	3 g

Whisk all dressing ingredients together and set aside. In a large salad bowl, toss together the salad ingredients. Add the dressing and toss to coat. Serve immediately.

Fresh Beet and Carrot Salad

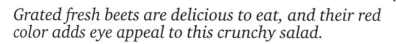

Total Servings: 6
Serving Size: 1 cup

Grated fresh beets are delicious to eat, and their red color adds eye appeal to this crunchy salad.

Salad

3 cups grated fresh beets (about 3–4 medium beets), peeled and uncooked

2 cups grated raw carrots, peeled

1 cup grated raw zucchini, unpeeled
Romaine lettuce leaves to line salad bowls or individual plates

Dressing

1/2 cup rice vinegar

2 Tbsp sesame oil

1 Tbsp grated ginger

1 Tbsp dry sherry
Fresh ground pepper and salt to taste

Exchanges	
2 Vegetable	
1 Fat	
Calories	95
Calories from Fat	42
Total Fat	5 g
Saturated Fat	1 g
Cholesterol	0 mg
Sodium	90 mg
Total Carbohydrate	12 g
Dietary Fiber	3 g
Sugars	8 g
Protein	2 g

1. In a large bowl, toss together the grated beets, carrots, and zucchini.

2. In a blender, combine the dressing ingredients. Add to the beets and toss well.

3. Place the romaine lettuce leaves on individual plates or in a large salad bowl. Pile on the beet mixture and serve.

Diabetic Meals in 30 Minutes—Or Less!

Broccoli Salad

Total Servings: 6
Serving Size: 1 cup

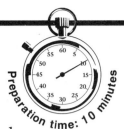

This broccoli salad goes very well with any Asian food.

Salad
- 2 quarts water
- 6 cups broccoli florets (about 2–3 lb)

Dressing
- 1 Tbsp corn oil
- 2 Tbsp sesame oil
- 3 Tbsp lite soy sauce
- 1/2 cup minced scallions
- 3 garlic cloves, minced

Exchanges	
1 Vegetable	
1 1/2 Fat	
Calories	95
Calories from Fat	66
Total Fat	7 g
Saturated Fat	1 g
Cholesterol	0 mg
Sodium	328 mg
Total Carbohydrate	6 g
Dietary Fiber	3 g
Sugars	3 g
Protein	3 g

1. In a large pot, bring the water to a boil. Add the broccoli and blanch for 2–3 minutes. Immediately drain the broccoli and then plunge it in a bowl of ice water to stop the cooking process. Drain again. Place in a large salad bowl.

2. Combine the dressing ingredients. Add it to the blanched broccoli and toss well. Refrigerate until ready to serve.

Healthy Coleslaw

Total Servings: 6
Serving Size: 1 cup

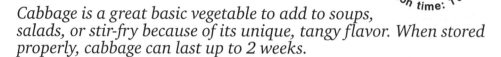

Cabbage is a great basic vegetable to add to soups, salads, or stir-fry because of its unique, tangy flavor. When stored properly, cabbage can last up to 2 weeks.

Salad

- 3 cups shredded green cabbage (1/2 medium head)
- 2 cups shredded red cabbage
- 1 cup shredded carrot
- 1/2 cup golden raisins

Dressing

- 1/3 cup reduced-fat mayonnaise
- 1/4 cup plain reduced-fat yogurt
- 2 Tbsp apple juice concentrate
- 2 Tbsp poppy seeds
- 2 Tbsp red wine vinegar

Exchanges	
1 Fruit	
1 Vegetable	
1 Fat	
Calories	135
Calories from Fat	52
Total Fat	6 g
Saturated Fat	1 g
Cholesterol	6 mg
Sodium	123 mg
Total Carbohydrate	19 g
Dietary Fiber	3 g
Sugars	15 g
Protein	3 g

1. Combine the cabbage, carrot, and raisins in a large bowl. Toss well.

2. Combine all the dressing ingredients. Add the dressing to the cabbage mixture and toss well. Refrigerate until ready to serve.

Diabetic Meals in 30 Minutes—Or Less!

Low-Fat Dijon Potato Salad

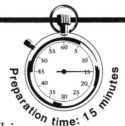

Total Servings: 6
Serving Size: 1/2 cup

Reduced-fat buttermilk and Dijon mustard give this salad a great flavor, but with much less fat!

Salad

- 1 lb red potatoes, unpeeled and cubed
- 1/2 cup diagonally sliced celery
- 1/4 cup sliced scallions
- 2 Tbsp chopped shallots

Dressing

- 1/2 cup reduced-fat buttermilk
- 2 Tbsp reduced-fat mayonnaise
- 1 Tbsp Dijon mustard
- 1 Tbsp tarragon vinegar

Exchanges	
1 Starch	
1/2 Fat	
Calories	97
Calories from Fat	17
Total Fat	2 g
Saturated Fat	0 g
Cholesterol	3 mg
Sodium	103 mg
Total Carbohydrate	18 g
Dietary Fiber	2 g
Sugars	3 g
Protein	2 g

1. In a medium-sized pot, cover the cubed potatoes with water. Bring to a boil, lower the heat, and cook on medium heat until potatoes are tender, yet firm (about 15 minutes).

2. Toss cooked potatoes with celery, scallions, and shallots.

3. In a small bowl, combine all dressing ingredients. Add to the potato salad and mix well. Refrigerate until ready to serve.

Coriander Carrot Salad

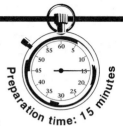

Total Servings: 6
Serving Size: 1 cup

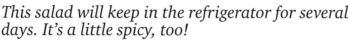

This salad will keep in the refrigerator for several days. It's a little spicy, too!

Salad

- 3 large carrots, peeled and grated
- 3 Tbsp chopped shallots
- 2 Tbsp minced parsley

Dressing

- 2 Tbsp olive oil
- 3 Tbsp fresh lemon juice
- 2 tsp cumin
- 1 Tbsp coriander seeds
- 1 tsp turmeric
  Dash cayenne pepper
  Fresh ground pepper to taste

Exchanges	
2 Vegetable	
1 Fat	
Calories	81
Calories from Fat	42
Total Fat	5 g
Saturated Fat	1 g
Cholesterol	0 mg
Sodium	32 mg
Total Carbohydrate	10 g
Dietary Fiber	3 g
Sugars	6 g
Protein	1 g

Combine the grated carrots, shallots, and parsley in a large salad bowl. Whisk together the dressing ingredients. Toss the dressing with the carrots. Refrigerate until ready to serve.

Diabetic Meals in 30 Minutes—Or Less!

Italian Bean Salad

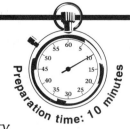

Total Servings: 6
Serving Size: 1/2 cup

Earthy balsamic vinegar dribbled over this hearty salad gives it a special flavor.

2	15-oz cans white beans, drained
1	small red onion, minced
3	stalks celery, diagonally sliced
1/4	cup sliced scallions
1/2	cup minced parsley
2	Tbsp balsamic vinegar
1	Tbsp olive oil
	Fresh ground pepper to taste

Exchanges
2 Starch

Calories	167
Calories from Fat	26
Total Fat	3 g
Saturated Fat	0 g
Cholesterol	0 mg
Sodium	188 mg
Total Carbohydrate	28 g
Dietary Fiber	5 g
Sugars	4 g
Protein	9 g

Combine all ingredients in the order given. Add more balsamic vinegar if desired. Refrigerate until ready to serve.

Fresh Snow Pea and Tri-Colored Pepper Salad

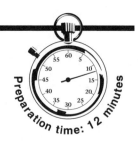

Total Servings: 6
Serving Size: about 1 cup

This salad is almost too pretty to eat.

Salad

    2 quarts water
    1 each small green, red, and yellow
       peppers, cored and sliced thin
1/4 lb fresh snow peas, trimmed
1/2 cup halved cherry tomatoes

Dressing

    3 Tbsp balsamic vinegar
    1 Tbsp minced shallot
    1 Tbsp olive oil
    2 tsp fresh lemon juice
    2 tsp Dijon mustard
      Fresh ground pepper and salt to taste

Exchanges
1 Vegetable
1/2 Fat
Calories...................... 55
Calories from Fat 23
Total Fat...................... 3 g
Saturated Fat .... 0 g
Cholesterol............. 0 mg
Sodium.................. 49 mg
Total Carbohydrate . 8 g
Dietary Fiber............ 2 g
Sugars .... 5 g
Protein...................... 2 g

1. In a large pot, bring the water to a boil. Add the sliced peppers and blanch for 2 minutes. Add the snow peas and blanch 30 seconds more. Drain. Plunge the peppers and snow peas into ice water to stop the cooking process. Drain again.

2. In a large salad bowl, toss the blanched peppers and snow peas with the cherry tomatoes.

3. Combine the dressing ingredients in a small bowl. Add the dressing to the pepper mixture and toss well. Refrigerate until ready to serve.

Sliced Tomatoes with Italian Parsley Dressing

Total Servings: 6
Serving Size: 1 cup

Preparation time: 10 minutes

This salad can be assembled right before serving.

Salad

 2–3 large, ripe salad tomatoes

Dressing

 1/2 cup minced Italian parsley
  2 Tbsp minced fresh basil
  3 Tbsp olive oil
  2 Tbsp lemon juice
  4 garlic cloves, minced
    Fresh ground pepper and salt to taste

Exchanges	
1 Vegetable	
1 1/2 Fat	
Calories	90
Calories from Fat	65
Total Fat	7 g
Saturated Fat	1 g
Cholesterol	0 mg
Sodium	38 mg
Total Carbohydrate	7 g
Dietary Fiber	2 g
Sugars	4 g
Protein	1 g

1. Slice the tomatoes and place them on a platter in an overlapping pattern.

2. In a blender or food processor, combine the dressing ingredients. Drizzle the dressing over the tomatoes just prior to serving.

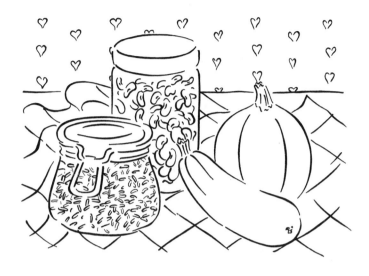

Vegetarian Fare

Vegetarian cooking is more sophisticated and interesting today than back in the hippie days of the 1960s! Eating vegetarian food has many benefits. The high-fiber content of most dishes makes them ideal to aid in weight control, and they're good for the digestive system, too. Grains and pastas are still relatively inexpensive and are well liked by almost everyone.

Try to purchase good pasta, such as imported Italian varieties made from hard durum semolina wheat; they cook up nice and firm and are tastier than American wheat. Look for whole-wheat varieties for a nuttier taste. Try brown rice instead of white for a bit more fiber and a much better flavor.

In these recipes, assume that the 1-cup serving size is for a main dish. To serve as a side dish, reduce the serving size to 1/2 cup.

Pick up a fork and dig into these nutritious, hearty, and delicious dishes!

TIPS FOR SUCCESS

CHINESE SESAME NOODLES

PASTA PUTTANESCA

RIGATONI WITH EGGPLANT AND MUSHROOMS

SHELLS AGLI OLIO

ANGEL HAIR PASTA WITH TOMATO SEAFOOD CREAM SAUCE

MOROCCAN COUSCOUS WITH CHICKPEAS

COUSCOUS TABOULI

VEGETABLE RICE AND BEANS

INDIAN RICE CURRY

TWO-TONE RICE PILAF

Tips for Success

Since brown rice does take longer to cook than white rice, follow these steps for preparing it and freezing it, so you will always have it on hand.

Prepare the rice by first rinsing it under water in a colander. Boil double the amount of liquid (water or broth) in a saucepan. Add your rinsed rice slowly to the pan, bring to a boil, cover, lower the heat, and cook for 45 minutes, until the water is absorbed. Do not stir while cooking—this loosens the starch and causes the grain to become very gummy.

Place the cooked rice in heavy-duty plastic zip-top bags (the 1-quart size is best) and freeze. When you're ready to use it, place the bag in the microwave. On the defrost setting, defrost rice for about 8 minutes, just until it breaks up. Then reheat the rice gently either in the microwave or on the stovetop until it's hot.

There are also couscous recipes included in this chapter. Couscous is very easy to work with. Simply rehydrate couscous in double the amount of liquid. It will rehydrate in as little as 5 minutes and is ready to go. Almost all supermarkets carry couscous.

You can also use canned beans in this chapter's recipes. Just thoroughly rinse the beans to remove excess salt. Beans are a great source of dietary fiber, too.

Chinese Sesame Noodles

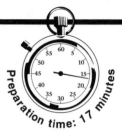

Total Servings: 6
Serving Size: 1 cup

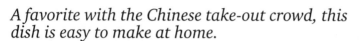

A favorite with the Chinese take-out crowd, this dish is easy to make at home.

1 Tbsp peanut butter
2 Tbsp lite soy sauce
1 tsp sesame oil
3 garlic cloves, minced
1 tsp grated ginger
2 cups cooked thin spaghetti noodles
1/2 cup thinly sliced red pepper
1/2 cup thinly sliced carrots
1/4 cup minced scallions
1/4 cup bean sprouts
    Red pepper flakes

Exchange	
1 Starch	
1/2 Fat	
Calories 102	
Calories from Fat 22	
Total Fat...................... 2 g	
Saturated Fat .... 0 g	
Cholesterol............... 0 mg	
Sodium .... 219 mg	
Total Carbohydrate 17 g	
Dietary Fiber............ 2 g	
Sugars .... 3 g	
Protein .... 3 g	

1. In a small saucepan, combine the peanut butter, soy sauce, sesame oil, garlic, and ginger. Bring the mixture to a boil, reduce the heat, and simmer for 3 minutes.

2. Combine the remaining ingredients and pour the hot peanut sesame dressing over the pasta vegetable mixture. Serve immediately or chill and serve cold.

Pasta Puttanesca

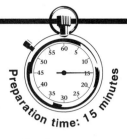

Total Servings: 6
Serving Size: 1 cup pasta with about 1/2 cup
vegetables and sauce

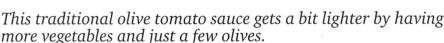

*This traditional olive tomato sauce gets a bit lighter by having
more vegetables and just a few olives.*

Sauce
  2 tsp olive oil
  1 medium onion, chopped
  4 garlic cloves, minced
  2 carrots, peeled and diced
  1 28-oz can plum tomatoes, coarsely
     chopped, undrained
  2 Tbsp white wine
  2 Tbsp minced basil
  2 Tbsp chopped black olives
  2 tsp capers

Pasta
  6 cups cooked fusilli (corkscrew) pasta

Garnish
  2 Tbsp minced parsley
  2 Tbsp grated Parmesan cheese

Exchanges	
3 Starch	
1 Vegetable	
Calories	276
Calories from Fat	32
Total Fat	4 g
Saturated Fat	1 g
Cholesterol	1 mg
Sodium	283 mg
Total Carbohydrate	52 g
Dietary Fiber	5 g
Sugars	8 g
Protein	9 g

1. In a heavy skillet over medium heat, heat the oil. Sauté the onion and garlic for 5 minutes. Add the carrots and continue to sauté for 5 more minutes.

2. Add the tomatoes and white wine and bring to a boil. Lower the heat and simmer for 15 minutes.

3. Add the basil, olives, and capers and simmer for 5 more minutes.

4. Toss the cooked fusilli with the sauce. Garnish with parsley and grated Parmesan cheese as desired.

Rigatoni with Eggplant and Mushrooms

Total Servings: 6
Serving Size: 1 cup pasta with about 2/3 cup vegetables and sauce

This very filling vegetarian dish needs only a salad and warm bread to complete it.

Sauce

- 1 Tbsp olive oil
- 1/4 cup dry white wine
- 3 garlic cloves, minced
- 1 red onion, chopped
- 1 cup diced eggplant, unpeeled
- 1 cup sliced mushrooms
- 1 28-oz can plum tomatoes, coarsely chopped, drained
- 2 tsp minced thyme
  Fresh ground pepper to taste

Pasta

- 6 cups cooked rigatoni pasta

Garnish

- 2 Tbsp grated Parmesan cheese

Exchanges	
2 Starch	
2 Vegetable	
1/2 Fat	
Calories	232
Calories from Fat	35
Total Fat	4 g
Saturated Fat	1 g
Cholesterol	1 mg
Sodium	178 mg
Total Carbohydrate	41 g
Dietary Fiber	4 g
Sugars	6 g
Protein	8 g

1. In a heavy skillet over medium heat, heat the oil and wine together. Add the garlic and onion and sauté for 5 minutes. Add the eggplant and sauté for 5 more minutes.

2. Add the mushrooms and sauté until mushrooms begin to brown, about 5 minutes. Add the plum tomatoes and bring to a boil. Lower the heat, cover, and simmer 10 minutes. Add the minced thyme and fresh ground pepper.

3. Toss the sauce with the cooked rigatoni. Top with Parmesan cheese.

Preparation time: 15 minutes

Shells Agli Olio

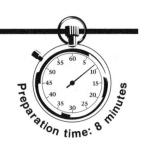

Preparation time: 8 minutes

Total Servings: 6
Serving Size: 1 cup

This is the simplest of all Italian sauces.

1/4 cup olive oil
2 Tbsp white wine
10 garlic cloves, minced
1 cup fresh spinach leaves, stems removed, torn into small pieces
1 lb cooked shell pasta

Exchanges	
2 1/2 Starch	
1 1/2 Fat	
Calories	256
Calories from Fat	89
Total Fat	10 g
Saturated Fat	1 g
Cholesterol	0 mg
Sodium	10 mg
Total Carbohydrate	35 g
Dietary Fiber	2 g
Sugars	3 g
Protein	6 g

1. In a heavy skillet, heat the oil and wine. Add the garlic and sauté for 5 minutes. Add the spinach and sauté just until it wilts.

2. Toss the garlic spinach sauce with the hot shells and serve.

Angel Hair Pasta with Tomato Seafood Cream Sauce

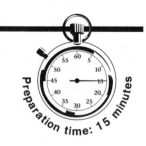

Preparation time: 15 minutes

Total Servings: 6
Serving Size: 1 cup with 2 oz seafood

Angel hair pasta is light and cooks quickly.

2	tsp olive oil
2	garlic cloves, minced
1	cup seeded, finely diced tomato
1 1/2	cups evaporated nonfat milk
1	tsp marjoram
	Fresh ground pepper to taste
3/4	lb sea scallops
6	cups cooked angel hair pasta

Exchanges	
3 Starch	
1 Very Lean Meat	
Calories	289
Calories from Fat	27
Total Fat	3 g
Saturated Fat	0 g
Cholesterol	21 mg
Sodium	169 mg
Total Carbohydrate	44 g
Dietary Fiber	2 g
Sugars	10 g
Protein	20 g

1. In a skillet over medium-high heat, heat the oil. Add the garlic and sauté for 30 seconds. Add the tomato and sauté for 2 minutes.

2. Add the evaporated milk and stir constantly over medium heat until thickened. Add the marjoram and pepper.

3. Add the scallops and cook for 2 minutes until the scallops turn opaque.

4. Pour the sauce over the angel hair pasta and serve.

Moroccan Couscous with Chickpeas

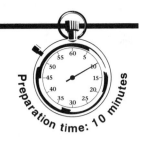

Preparation time: 10 minutes

Total Servings: 6
Serving Size: 1 cup

Using couscous is the fastest way to get a good main dish on the table in minutes. No stovetop is required—just rehydrate the couscous and eat!

Couscous

2 cups dry couscous, rehydrated (To rehydrate, pour 4 cups boiling water over the couscous in a heat-proof bowl. Let stand for 5 minutes until the water is absorbed.)

1 cup canned chickpeas (garbanzo beans), drained

1/4 cup minced parsley

2 Tbsp minced scallions

Dressing

1/4 cup fresh lemon juice

2 Tbsp olive oil

1 Tbsp cumin

1 tsp coriander

1 tsp paprika

1/2 tsp cayenne pepper

2 garlic cloves, minced

Exchanges	
4 Starch	
Calories	320
Calories from Fat	51
Total Fat	6 g
Saturated Fat	1 g
Cholesterol	0 mg
Sodium	50 mg
Total Carbohydrate	56 g
Dietary Fiber	5 g
Sugars	3 g
Protein	10 g

1. In a bowl, combine the couscous, chickpeas, parsley, and scallions.

2. Combine all dressing ingredients and pour over the couscous and chickpeas. Serve at room temperature or refrigerate until ready to serve.

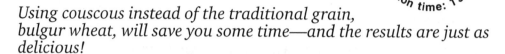

Couscous Tabouli

Total Servings: 6
Serving Size: 1 cup

Using couscous instead of the traditional grain, bulgur wheat, will save you some time—and the results are just as delicious!

Couscous

1 1/2 cups dry couscous, rehydrated (To rehydrate, pour 4 cups boiling water over the couscous in a heat-proof bowl. Let stand for 5 minutes until the water is absorbed.)
2 medium tomatoes, chopped
4 scallions, chopped
1/2 cup diced cucumber
1 cup minced parsley

Dressing

1/4 cup lemon juice
2 Tbsp olive oil
1 tsp cumin
Fresh ground pepper and salt to taste

Exchanges	
2 1/2 Starch	
1 Vegetable	
1/2 Fat	
Calories	233
Calories from Fat	46
Total Fat	5 g
Saturated Fat	1 g
Cholesterol	0 mg
Sodium	42 mg
Total Carbohydrate	40 g
Dietary Fiber	4 g
Sugars	3 g
Protein	7 g

1. Combine the rehydrated couscous with the tomatoes, scallions, cucumber, and parsley.

2. Whisk together the dressing ingredients.

3. Pour dressing over the couscous and serve or refrigerate until serving time.

Diabetic Meals in 30 Minutes—Or Less!

Vegetable Rice and Beans

Total Servings: 6
Serving Size: 1 cup

This is a quick skillet dish to whip up with ingredients you probably have on hand. Precook white or brown rice to save time and keep covered in a container in the refrigerator. Brown rice will take longer to cook, so be sure to have some prepared beforehand.

2 tsp olive oil
1 medium onion, chopped
3 cloves garlic, minced
2 medium tomatoes, finely diced
1 carrot, peeled and diced
1 15-oz can red kidney beans
1 tsp minced thyme
Fresh ground pepper to taste
4 cups cooked white or brown rice

Exchanges	
3 Starch	
Calories	248
Calories from Fat	29
Total Fat	3 g
Saturated Fat	1 g
Cholesterol	0 mg
Sodium	277 mg
Total Carbohydrate	48 g
Dietary Fiber	6 g
w/white rice	4 g
Sugars	6 g
Protein	8 g

1. In a heavy skillet over medium heat, heat the oil. Add the onion and garlic and sauté for 5 minutes.

2. Add the tomatoes and carrot and cook for 5–8 more minutes. Add the kidney beans and thyme and simmer for 5 minutes. Grind in pepper.

3. Pour the vegetable bean mixture over hot cooked rice and serve.

Indian Rice Curry

Total Servings: 6
Serving Size: 1 cup

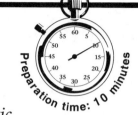

Having cooked rice on hand means this aromatic dish can be ready fast.

2 tsp olive oil
1 small onion, minced
1/4 cup chopped tart apple
2 tsp curry powder
Dash cayenne pepper
4 cups cooked white or brown rice
2 cups canned chickpeas, drained
1 Tbsp fresh lemon juice
Fresh ground pepper to taste

Exchanges	
3 Starch	
Calories	257
Calories from Fat	37
Total Fat	4 g
Saturated Fat	1 g
Cholesterol	0 mg
Sodium	86 mg
Total Carbohydrate	47 g
Dietary Fiber	5 g
w/white rice	3 g
Sugars	5 g
Protein	8 g

1. In a heavy skillet over medium heat, heat the oil. Add the onion and sauté for 3 minutes. Add the apple and sauté for 3 more minutes. Add the curry powder and cayenne to coat the apple and onion.

2. Add the cooked rice and chickpeas. Cook through until rice and beans are hot. Sprinkle with lemon juice, add pepper to taste, and serve.

Diabetic Meals in 30 Minutes—Or Less!

Two-Tone Rice Pilaf

Total Servings: 6
Serving Size: 1 cup

Here, have the best of both worlds: fluffy white rice and nutty brown rice team up in this Italian-flavored dish.

Preparation time: 15 minutes

2 tsp olive oil	
1 medium onion, minced	
4 garlic cloves, minced	
2 scallions, minced	
4 plum tomatoes, chopped	
1 cup sliced asparagus	
1/2 cup low-fat, reduced-sodium chicken broth	
2 Tbsp fresh minced basil	
1 tsp fresh minced oregano	
1/2 cup sliced rehydrated sun-dried tomatoes	
2 cups each cooked brown and white rice	
Fresh ground pepper to taste	

Exchanges
2 1/2 Starch

Calories	203
Calories from Fat	27
Total Fat	3 g
Saturated Fat	1 g
Cholesterol	0 mg
Sodium	99 mg
Total Carbohydrate	40 g
Dietary Fiber	4 g
Sugars	5 g
Protein	6 g

1. In a heavy skillet, heat the oil. Add the onion and garlic and sauté for 5 minutes. Add the scallions and sauté 1 minute.

2. Add the tomatoes, asparagus, and chicken broth. Cover the pan and let steam for 3–4 minutes.

3. Add the basil, oregano, and sun-dried tomatoes. Simmer for 5 minutes.

4. Add the cooked rices and toss well. Serve.

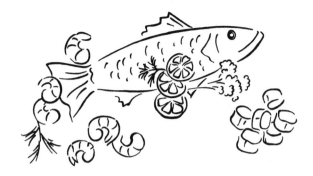

THE DAILY CATCH

Most people probably have fond memories of the only fish dish they ate as children: frozen breaded fishsticks! Today there are so many varieties of fresh fish that it is hard to resist preparing it in new and delicious ways.

Here are a few pointers on selecting fish:

- Try to go to a fish market that you are familiar with. This way you will know their delivery schedule and can be assured of the freshest fish possible.

- Look for steaks and fillets that appear to be freshly cut, without a dried or brown look. A mushy flesh may indicate that the fish has been defrosted and refrozen.

- Plan your menus carefully. Fresh fish should be used within 24 hours for the best taste and freshness. Keep fresh fish on ice in your refrigerator to keep it at its best. If you must freeze your fish, wrap the fish well and try to use it within 1–3 months.

- Be gentle when you cook fish! Fish is done when it just turns opaque. If it overflakes, it is overcooked! When cooking shellfish, such as shrimp, cook it until it just turns pink and then remove it from the heat. Scallops should be cooked just until they turn opaque, about 1–2 minutes.

So bait your line and throw it in—it's time for some great fish!

Swordfish with Fresh Tomato Sauce

Broiled Crab Cakes

Tandoori Shrimp

Steamed Oriental Sole

Grilled Salmon with Rice Vinegar Splash

Shrimp Fra Diablo

Halibut in Foil

Ginger and Lime Salmon

Mediterranean Seafood Pasta

Asian Tuna Steaks

Swordfish with Fresh Tomato Sauce

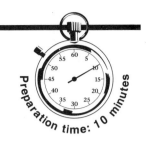

Preparation time: 10 minutes

Total Servings: 6
Serving Size: 3 oz fish and sauce

Keep swordfish juicy and moist with this fresh-from-the-vine tomato sauce.

Fish
1 1/2 lb swordfish steaks
   2 Tbsp fresh lemon juice
   1 Tbsp olive oil

Sauce
 1/4 cup white wine
   3 garlic cloves, minced
   2 scallions, chopped
   4 ripe tomatoes, chopped
   2 tsp minced thyme

Exchanges	
1 Vegetable	
3 Very Lean Meat	
1 Fat	
Calories	178
Calories from Fat	54
Total Fat	6 g
Saturated Fat	1 g
Cholesterol	44 mg
Sodium	113 mg
Total Carbohydrate	6 g
Dietary Fiber	1 g
Sugars	4 g
Protein	23 g

1. Marinate the fish in the lemon juice and olive oil for 10 minutes at room temperature while you prepare the tomato sauce.

2. In a heavy skillet, heat the wine. When it is slightly boiling, add the garlic and scallions. Sauté for 3 minutes. Add the tomatoes and thyme. Bring to a boil and simmer for 5 minutes.

3. Remove the swordfish from the marinade. Grill or broil the swordfish for 3–4 minutes per side. Top with the fresh tomato sauce to serve.

Broiled Crab Cakes

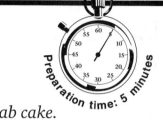

Total Servings: 6
Serving Size: 3 oz

Nothing hits the spot like a simple broiled crab cake.

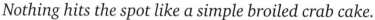

1 1/2 lb backfin crabmeat, cartilage and
     shells removed
2 Tbsp reduced-fat mayonnaise
2 Tbsp Dijon mustard
3 Tbsp minced onion
1 egg
    Dash Tabasco® sauce

Exchanges	
3 Very Lean Meat	
1/2 Fat	
Calories	131
Calories from Fat	38
Total Fat	4 g
Saturated Fat	1 g
Cholesterol	132 mg
Sodium	375 mg
Total Carbohydrate	1 g
Dietary Fiber	0 g
Sugars	1 g
Protein	20 g

Combine all ingredients and shape into six patties. Broil 6 inches
from heat source, 3 minutes per side, until golden brown. Serve
immediately.

Tandoori Shrimp

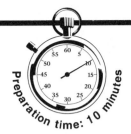

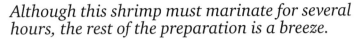

Total Servings: 6
Serving Size: 4 oz

Although this shrimp must marinate for several hours, the rest of the preparation is a breeze.

3	Tbsp coarsely chopped ginger
1	medium onion, coarsely chopped
6	garlic cloves
1/4	cup olive oil
1 1/4	cup plain low- or nonfat yogurt
2	Tbsp ground cumin
1	tsp turmeric
2	tsp paprika
1	tsp cayenne pepper
1 1/2	lb shelled and deveined large shrimp

Exchanges

3 Lean Meat

Calories	172
Calories from Fat	60
Total Fat	7 g
Saturated Fat	1 g
Cholesterol	171 mg
Sodium	175 mg
Total Carbohydrate	3 g
Dietary Fiber	0 g
Sugars	3 g
Protein	24 g

1. Combine all marinade ingredients in a food processor or blender. Marinate the shrimp for 4 hours.

2. Grill the shrimp for 3 minutes, about 6 inches from the heat source.

Steamed Oriental Sole

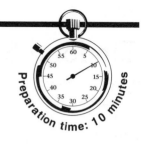

Total Servings: 6
Serving Size: 3 oz

This fish has an elegant flavor, but is still simple to prepare.

2 scallions, cut diagonally into 1-inch pieces
2 carrots, peeled and julienned
1 cup finely chopped bok choy cabbage
1 cup fresh snow peas, trimmed
4 thin slices fresh ginger, julienned
1 1/2 lb sole fillets
3 Tbsp lite soy sauce
1 Tbsp sesame oil
2 Tbsp dry sherry

Exchanges	
1 Vegetable	
3 Very Lean Meat	
1/2 Fat	
Calories	164
Calories from Fat	33
Total Fat	4 g
Saturated Fat	1 g
Cholesterol	60 mg
Sodium	429 mg
Total Carbohydrate	8 g
Dietary Fiber	2 g
Sugars	4 g
Protein	23 g

1. Prepare the vegetables and ginger. Place the sole fillets on a large heat-proof plate. Scatter all of the vegetables and the ginger over the sole fillets.

2. Combine the soy sauce, sesame oil, and sherry. Sprinkle the sauce over the vegetables and fish.

3. Place a steamer rack in a large wok or saucepot. Pour 3 inches of water into the bottom of the wok or pot. Place the plate of fish and vegetables on the steamer rack.

4. Cover and let steam on high heat for 5–8 minutes. Add more water to the bottom of the wok or pot if necessary. Remove fish and vegetables and serve.

Grilled Salmon with Rice Vinegar Splash

Total Servings: 6
Serving Size: 3 oz

The secret to this dish is splashing a very simple rice vinegar sauce on the salmon fillets just after you remove them from the broiler.

Sauce
- 1 cup rice vinegar
- 3 cloves garlic, minced
- 3 shallots, finely minced
- 3 slices ginger, minced

Salmon
- 1 1/2 lb salmon fillets
- 1 Tbsp olive oil

Garnish
- Sprigs of parsley or cilantro

Exchanges	
1 Vegetable	
3 Lean Meat	
1/2 Fat	
Calories	220
Calories from Fat	108
Total Fat	12 g
Saturated Fat	2 g
Cholesterol	77 mg
Sodium	60 mg
Total Carbohydrate	3 g
Dietary Fiber	0 g
Sugars	2 g
Protein	24 g

1. Combine all sauce ingredients and set aside.

2. Brush each salmon fillet with a little olive oil. Broil 6 inches from the heat source for 3–4 minutes per side until done.

3. Splash the sauce over the cooked salmon fillets. Garnish with parsley or cilantro.

Shrimp Fra Diablo

Total Servings: 6
Serving Size: 3 oz shrimp plus sauce

Preparation time: 15 minutes

"Fra diablo" means a spicy tomato sauce. Serve this dish with pasta to cool it off a bit.

1	Tbsp olive oil
3	garlic cloves, minced
1	medium onion, chopped
1	15-oz can tomato puree
1	6-oz can tomato paste
2	Tbsp red wine
2	tsp crushed red pepper
2	tsp capers
2	Tbsp minced basil
1 1/2	lb shelled and deveined medium shrimp

Exchanges

1 Starch
3 Very Lean Meat

Calories	205
Calories from Fat	42
Total Fat	5 g
Saturated Fat	1 g
Cholesterol	170 mg
Sodium	299 mg
Total Carbohydrate	16 g
Dietary Fiber	3 g
Sugars	8 g
Protein	25 g

1. In a heavy skillet, heat the oil. Add the garlic and onion and sauté for 5 minutes. Add the tomato puree and tomato paste. Bring to a boil.

2. Add the red wine, red pepper, capers, and basil. Lower the heat and simmer for 15 minutes.

3. Add the shrimp and cook over low heat for 4–5 minutes, until the shrimp just turn pink. Serve over pasta if desired.

Halibut in Foil

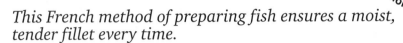

Total Servings: 6
Serving Size: 3–4 oz

This French method of preparing fish ensures a moist,
tender fillet every time.

2	tsp olive oil
6	4-oz halibut steaks
1/2	cup dry white wine
6	thyme sprigs
6	thin lemon slices
1 1/2	tsp fennel seeds
6	parsley sprigs
	Fresh ground pepper to taste

Exchanges
4 Very Lean Meat

Calories 144
  Calories from Fat 37
Total Fat .... 4 g
  Saturated Fat .... 1 g
Cholesterol .... 36 mg
Sodium .... 62 mg
Total Carbohydrate . 0 g
  Dietary Fiber .... 0 g
  Sugars .... 0 g
Protein .... 24 g

1. Preheat the oven to 350°F. Tear aluminum foil into six large
    squares. Brush each square with some olive oil.

2. Place the halibut in the center of the square. Drizzle each steak
    with some of the wine. Put a thyme sprig, a lemon slice, a few
    fennel seeds, and a parsley sprig on each piece of fish.

3. Grind pepper over each piece of fish. Seal the foil into a packet.
    Place all packets on a baking sheet and bake for 10–15 minutes.
    Place a packet on each plate and let each person carefully open it.
    Pour all juices on top of the fish.

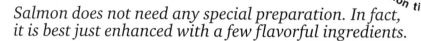

Ginger and Lime Salmon

Total Servings: 6
Serving Size: 3 oz

Salmon does not need any special preparation. In fact, it is best just enhanced with a few flavorful ingredients.

1 Tbsp sesame oil
1 Tbsp lite soy sauce
1 Tbsp grated ginger
2 Tbsp dry sherry
6 4-oz salmon fillets
1 Tbsp grated lime peel
1 Tbsp minced scallions
12 lime wedges

Exchanges	
3 Lean Meat	
1/2 Fat	
Calories	205
Calories from Fat	98
Total Fat	11 g
Saturated Fat	2 g
Cholesterol	77 mg
Sodium	109 mg
Total Carbohydrate	1 g
Dietary Fiber	0 g
Sugars	0 g
Protein	24 g

1. Mix together the sesame oil, soy sauce, ginger, and sherry. Sprinkle over the salmon and let it marinate for 15 minutes.

2. Prepare to steam. Fill the bottom of a large wok or saucepot with 3 inches of water. Place a steamer rack in the wok or pot. Place the fish fillets on a heat-proof plate. Cover the wok or pot and steam the fish for 10 minutes, until it is tender.

3. Sprinkle the fish with lime peel and scallions. Serve with lime wedges.

Mediterranean Seafood Pasta

Total Servings: 6
Serving Size: 1 cup cooked pasta with 3 1/2 oz seafood

The fruits of the sea enliven this European-inspired dish.

2 tsp olive oil
1 medium onion, minced
1 medium carrot, diced
1/2 cup each diced red and green peppers
1 1/2 cups crushed canned tomatoes
3 Tbsp dry white wine
2 tsp dried oregano
1 tsp dried or fresh chopped thyme
2 Tbsp lemon juice
1 lb shelled and deveined medium shrimp
1/2 lb sea scallops
6 cups cooked, shaped pasta (use rigatoni, penne, or shells)

Exchanges	
3 Starch	
2 Very Lean Meat	
Calories	315
Calories from Fat	31
Total Fat	3 g
Saturated Fat	1 g
Cholesterol	125 mg
Sodium	386 mg
Total Carbohydrate	43 g
Dietary Fiber	4 g
Sugars	7 g
Protein	26 g

1. In a large skillet, heat the oil. Add the onion and carrot and sauté for 5 minutes. Add the peppers and sauté for 3 more minutes.

2. Add the crushed tomatoes, wine, oregano, thyme, and lemon juice. Bring to a boil. Simmer for 10 minutes.

3. Add the seafood and cook over medium heat for 5 minutes until shrimp have turned pink and scallops are no longer translucent.

4. Place 3 1/2 oz of the seafood and sauce over each serving of pasta.

Asian Tuna Steaks

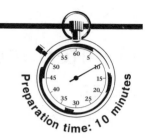

Total Servings: 6
Serving Size: 3–4 oz

Serve these tender steaks with Broccoli Salad
(see p. 49) for a delicious meal.

Marinade

- 1/4 cup orange juice (fresh or frozen)
- 2 Tbsp sesame oil
- 2 tsp sesame seeds
- 3 Tbsp lite soy sauce
- 1 Tbsp fresh grated ginger (or use 2 tsp ground ginger)
- 3 Tbsp chopped scallions

Tuna

1 1/2 lb tuna steaks

Exchanges	
3 Lean Meat	
Calories	184
Calories from Fat	71
Total Fat	8 g
Saturated Fat	2 g
Cholesterol	42
Sodium	194 mg
Total Carbohydrate	1 g
Dietary Fiber	0 g
Sugars	1 g
Protein	26 g

1. In a stainless steel bowl or plastic zip-top bag, combine all marinade ingredients. Add the tuna and let it marinate for 20 minutes.

2. Broil or grill the tuna 6 inches from the heat source for 4–5 minutes per side. Cook until done as desired (some people prefer their tuna more rare than others do).

Diabetic Meals in 30 Minutes—Or Less!

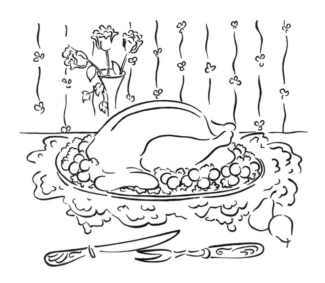

PERFECT POULTRY

Poultry is a great low-fat, high-protein food! Stick with white meat from chicken and turkey breasts—dark meat from chicken and turkey, as well as any part of goose and duck, is too high in fat and should be reserved for special occasions. Whole chickens and Cornish game hens are delicious, but can take a long time to prepare. Recently, free-range chicken has become an excellent, healthy option for poultry lovers—it's more expensive, but the meat is even lower in fat than regular chicken and has a tender, delicious flavor. Try to buy ground turkey from a butcher who grinds his or her own meat—most commercially prepared ground turkey contains a lot of dark meat and skin.

The first step in creating juicy, mouth-watering recipes is to always buy chicken and turkey with the skin attached. This fat layer keeps the meat moist and makes the final dish juicier. You should still remove the skin from the meat before cooking it—3 ounces of chicken skin has 40 grams of fat. It's also easy to make tasty chicken by marinating it. Marinating ensures that the tougher meat fibers are broken down, and it yields juicy, tender meat. Cooking it quickly also helps ensure tenderness.

SOUTH-OF-THE-BORDER CHICKEN WITH VARIATIONS

"WOK" THIS WAY

CHICKEN STIR-FRY WITH VEGETABLES

CRUNCHY CHICKEN WITH ASPARAGUS

SPICY CHICKEN WITH PEPPERS

SOUTHWESTERN CHICKEN SALAD

CURRIED CHICKEN SALAD WITH GRAPES

CHICKEN TARRAGON SALAD

CHICKEN AND GRAPES

BOMBAY CHICKEN

CHICKEN PAPRIKASH

CHICKEN MARSALA

TURKEY BURRITOS

GRILLED TURKEY WITH GARLIC SAUCE

TURKEY PROVENÇAL

STUFFED ZUCCHINI BOATS

South-of-the-Border Chicken with Variations

Total Servings: 6
Serving Size: 3–4 oz

This recipe provides several different marinades so you can cook variations of this delicious dish. (See pages 86–87 for microwave directions and marinade variations.)

Marinade

- 1/2 cup fresh lime juice
- 1 Tbsp olive oil
- 1/2 cup chopped yellow onion
- 1/2 cup chopped red pepper
- 2 garlic cloves, minced
- 2 Tbsp minced cilantro
- 1 Tbsp fresh minced oregano (or 1 tsp dried oregano)

Chicken

- 3 whole chicken breasts, skinned, boned, and halved

Garnish

Lime slices

Exchanges	
4 Very Lean Meat	
Calories	155
Calories from Fat	38
Total Fat	4 g
Saturated Fat	1 g
Cholesterol	73 mg
Sodium	64 mg
Total Carbohydrate	1 g
Dietary Fiber	0 g
Sugars	0 g
Protein	27 g

1. In a large bowl, combine all marinade ingredients. Add the chicken breasts and marinate for at least 2–3 hours, or up to 2 days.

2. To cook, drain marinade. Add the chicken breast halves to a broiler pan and set the oven rack 6 inches from the heat source or place the chicken on a hot outside grill with the grill rack set 6 inches above the heat source. Grill the chicken for 7–8 minutes per side until no trace of pink remains.

3. Garnish with lime slices and serve.

Marinade Variations

Follow the above directions for South-of-the-Border Chicken, except try one of these different marinades. All of these marinades will coat enough for three whole chicken breasts (about 21–23 oz). All marinades have the same nutritional analysis except the Rice Vinegar marinade, which has 116 mg of sodium.

Balsamic Mustard
1/4 cup low-fat, reduced-sodium chicken broth
  2 garlic cloves, minced
1/2 cup balsamic vinegar
  3 Tbsp Dijon mustard
  1 Tbsp olive oil
  1 Tbsp minced scallions

Herb Marinade
  2 Tbsp minced parsley
  2 tsp fresh minced thyme
  2 tsp fresh rosemary
  2 sage leaves
  1 tsp fresh minced tarragon
1/3 cup sherry vinegar
  1 Tbsp olive oil
    Fresh ground pepper to taste

Rice Vinegar
1/2 cup rice vinegar
  2 Tbsp dry sherry
  1 Tbsp sesame oil
  3 garlic cloves, minced
  1 Tbsp lite soy sauce
    Ground white pepper

Orange Cumin

- 1/4 cup fresh orange juice
- 1 Tbsp olive oil
- 2 tsp grated orange peel
- 1 tsp cumin
- 2 tsp minced parsley
- 2 Tbsp white wine

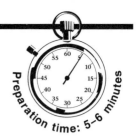

Lemon Pepper

- 1/2 cup dry white wine
- 1 Tbsp olive oil
- 1/3 cup low-fat, reduced-sodium chicken broth
- 1/4 cup lemon juice
- 2 tsp grated lemon peel
- 1 garlic clove, minced
- 1 Tbsp whole black peppercorns

Raspberry Shallot

- 1/2 cup raspberry vinegar
- 1 Tbsp olive oil
- 3 Tbsp minced shallots
- 2 tsp minced thyme
  Fresh ground pepper to taste

Microwave Directions

If you prefer to microwave your chicken, marinate the chicken as above. Arrange the chicken on a trivet in a baking dish big enough to accommodate all of the chicken. Put the meatier portions facing the walls of the microwave. Cover the chicken with waxed paper and cook on full power (high) for about 14 minutes, until juices run clear. Let stand for 4 minutes, covered. Garnish with lime slices.

"Wok" This Way

Using a wok can help you get dinner on the table fast. Here are some tips for foolproof wok cooking and several easy, delicious recipes to make.

- There are many woks to choose from. Buy one that suits your needs. It is preferable to purchase a non-electric wok. Woks created for the stove tend to be deeper and are better made than electric woks.

- Season your wok well. A properly seasoned wok will provide many years of cooking pleasure. Read the manufacturer's directions carefully for correct seasoning methods.

- Your stirring spoon should have a long handle and preferably have a flat edge. This will help with the fast hand motion necessary to stir-fry properly.

- Heat your wok without anything in it just a few seconds prior to beginning the recipe. This will prevent food from sticking to the wok.

- When adding food to the wok, make sure your ingredients are not ice cold. Bring meat, poultry, and fish up to room temperature prior to placing them in the wok. Otherwise, food will stick to the wok.

- Assemble all of your ingredients first and then proceed to stir-fry. Stir-frying is a very quick process and all ingredients need to be washed, chopped, and sliced so they are ready to go.

Diabetic Meals in 30 Minutes—Or Less!

Chicken Stir-Fry with Vegetables

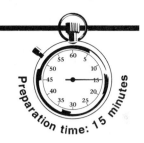

Total Servings: 6
Serving Size: 1 cup with 3 oz chicken

No oil is used to prepare this extremely tender chicken.

3	chicken breasts, halved, boned, and skinned
1	egg white, beaten
1	Tbsp cornstarch or arrowroot powder
3	Tbsp low-fat, reduced-sodium chicken broth
1/2	cup sliced mushrooms
2	small zucchini, cut into strips, unpeeled
1	cup fresh snow peas, trimmed
1/2	cup sliced scallions
1	Tbsp lite soy sauce

Exchanges
1 Vegetable
4 Very Lean Meat

Calories	171
Calories from Fat	29
Total Fat	3 g
Saturated Fat	1 g
Cholesterol	73 mg
Sodium	180 mg
Total Carbohydrate	5 g
Dietary Fiber	2 g
Sugars	2 g
Protein	29 g

1. Flatten each breast of chicken by placing it between two pieces of waxed paper and pounding it with a meat mallet. Pound until the breast is 1/4 inch thick. Cut into bite-size pieces.

2. Place chicken in a bowl. Add the egg white and cornstarch or arrowroot powder. Stir thoroughly. Let the chicken sit for 10 minutes and prepare all the vegetables.

3. Heat the broth in the wok. Add the chicken and stir-fry until it turns opaque, about 5–6 minutes. Remove the chicken from the wok.

4. Add the mushrooms to the wok and stir-fry for 2 minutes. Add the zucchini, snow peas, scallions, and soy sauce. Cover the pan and steam for 2 minutes. Add the chicken back to the wok and steam for 1 more minute.

Crunchy Chicken with Asparagus

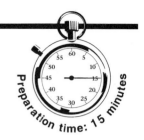

Preparation time: 15 minutes

Total Servings: 6
Serving Size: 1 cup with 3–4 oz chicken

The asparagus in this dish should remain bright green. Asparagus is best when it is crisp.

2 tsp peanut oil
2 Tbsp low-fat, reduced-sodium
  chicken broth
3 cloves garlic, minced
2 Tbsp minced scallions
3 chicken breasts, boned, skinned,
  halved, and cubed into 2-inch
  pieces
1 medium carrot, sliced thin
2 cups sliced asparagus (slice into
  2-inch pieces)
1/2 cup water chestnuts
2 Tbsp lite soy sauce
2 Tbsp white wine vinegar
1 tsp sesame oil
1/4 cup low-fat, reduced-sodium chicken
  broth
1 Tbsp cornstarch or arrowroot powder

Exchanges	
1 Vegetable	
4 Very Lean Meat	
1/2 Fat	
Calories	200
Calories from Fat	51
Total Fat	6 g
Saturated Fat	1 g
Cholesterol	73 mg
Sodium	289 mg
Total Carbohydrate	8 g
Dietary Fiber	2 g
Sugars	3 g
Protein	29 g

1. In a wok over medium-high heat, heat the oil and broth. Add the garlic and scallions and sauté for 30 seconds. Add the chicken and stir-fry for 5–8 minutes until it is opaque.

2. Push the chicken up on the sides of the wok. Add a little broth, if necessary, and add the carrot. Stir-fry for 2 minutes. Add the asparagus and stir-fry for 3 minutes. Add the water chestnuts and stir-fry 2 more minutes. Add chicken back to the center of the wok.

3. Combine the last five ingredients and mix until smooth. Add the sauce to the wok. Stir, cover, and steam for 2 minutes.

Spicy Chicken with Peppers

Total Servings: 6
Serving Size: 1 cup (3 oz chicken)

Preparation time: 15 minutes

This dish is not for the faint hearted. However, use fewer chili peppers if you want to tone down the heat.

1 Tbsp peanut oil
3 garlic cloves, minced
3 small red chili peppers, minced
3 chicken breasts, boned, skinned, halved, and cut into 2-inch pieces
2 Tbsp low-fat, reduced-sodium chicken broth
1 each small red and green pepper, sliced thin
1 cup sliced celery
1/2 cup sliced scallions
1 Tbsp lite soy sauce

Exchanges	
1 Vegetable	
4 Very Lean Meat	
1/2 Fat	
Calories	190
Calories from Fat	50
Total Fat	6 g
Saturated Fat	1 g
Cholesterol	73 mg
Sodium	185 mg
Total Carbohydrate	7 g
Dietary Fiber	1 g
Sugars	3 g
Protein	28 g

1. In a wok, heat the oil over medium-high heat. Add the garlic and chili peppers and stir-fry for 30 seconds. Do not let the mixture burn.

2. Add the chicken and stir-fry for 5–8 minutes until it is opaque. Push the chicken up on the sides of the wok.

3. Add the chicken broth to the wok. Stir-fry the peppers for 4 minutes. Add the celery and scallions and stir-fry for 2 minutes.

4. Push the chicken back to the center of the wok. Add the soy sauce. Cover and steam for 2 minutes.

Southwestern Chicken Salad

Total Servings: 6
Serving Size: 1 cup

Preparation time: 10 minutes

You can also omit the chicken from this recipe for a high-fiber, vegetarian bean and corn salad (the nutritional analysis for this variation is in parentheses, and the yield is four 1-cup servings).

Salad

  1 cup cooked corn kernels
  1 cup diced tomatoes
  1 cup frozen green peas, thawed
1/2 cup each sliced red and green
    pepper
1/3 cup canned black beans, drained
  2 cups cooked, cubed chicken
    breast

Dressing

  1 Tbsp olive oil
1/4 cup lime juice
  2 tsp cumin
  1 Tbsp chopped cilantro
  2 tsp chili powder
  1 tsp oregano

Exchanges	
1 (1 1/2) Starch	
2 (0) Very Lean Meat	
1/2 (1/2) Fat	
Calories	181 (137)
Calories from Fat	55 (36)
Total Fat	6 g (4 g)
Saturated Fat	1 g (1 g)
Cholesterol	42 mg (0 mg)
Sodium	94 mg (80 mg)
Total Carbohydrate	16 g (23 g)
Dietary Fiber	4 g (6 g)
Sugars	4 g (6 g)
Protein	17 g (5 g)

Combine all salad ingredients. In a blender or food processor, blend all dressing ingredients. Toss the dressing with the salad and serve.

Curried Chicken Salad with Grapes

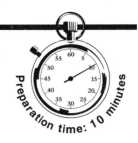

Total Servings: 6
Serving Size: 1 cup

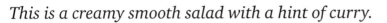

This is a creamy smooth salad with a hint of curry.

Salad

3	cups cooked, cubed chicken breasts
1 1/2	cups halved green or red grapes
1/2	cup sliced celery
2	Tbsp sliced scallions
1/2	cup diced red pepper

Dressing

3/4	cup reduced-fat mayonnaise
2	Tbsp orange juice
1	tsp curry powder
	Fresh ground pepper to taste

Exchanges	
1/2 Carbohydrate	
4 Lean Meat	
Calories	273
Calories from Fat	112
Total Fat	12 g
Saturated Fat	2 g
Cholesterol	84 mg
Sodium	293 mg
Total Carbohydrate	10 g
Dietary Fiber	1 g
Sugars	8 g
Protein	27 g

Combine all salad ingredients. Combine all dressing ingredients in a small bowl and whisk together until smooth. Toss the dressing with the salad and serve.

Chicken Tarragon Salad

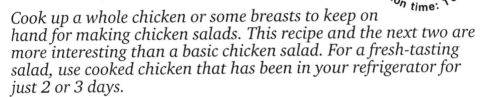

Total Servings: 6
Serving Size: 1 cup

Cook up a whole chicken or some breasts to keep on hand for making chicken salads. This recipe and the next two are more interesting than a basic chicken salad. For a fresh-tasting salad, use cooked chicken that has been in your refrigerator for just 2 or 3 days.

Salad

- 3 cups cooked, cubed chicken breast
- 1 cup sliced celery
- 1 cup diced onion
- 1/2 cup diced zucchini, unpeeled

Dressing

- 3/4 cup fat-free mayonnaise
- 2 Tbsp fat-free sour cream
- 2 Tbsp minced tarragon
- 1 Tbsp minced parsley
- Fresh ground pepper to taste

Exchanges	
1/2 Carbohydrate	
3 Very Lean Meat	
Calories	156
Calories from Fat	24
Total Fat	3 g
Saturated Fat	0.7 g
Cholesterol	60 mg
Sodium	288 mg
Total Carbohydrate	8 g
Dietary Fiber	1 g
Sugars	4 g
Protein	23 g

Combine all salad ingredients. Combine all dressing ingredients in a small bowl and whisk together until smooth. Toss the dressing with the salad and serve.

Chicken and Grapes

Total Servings: 6
Serving Size: 3–4 oz

This is the French-inspired recipe Chicken Veronique, without the cream or butter.

3   whole chicken breasts, boned,
      skinned, and halved, pounded until
      1/4 inch thick
1/3   cup unbleached white flour
      Fresh ground pepper and salt to taste
2   tsp canola oil
1   small onion, minced
1   cup low-fat, reduced-sodium chicken
      broth
3   Tbsp low-sugar orange marmalade
2   tsp fresh minced rosemary
2   tsp lemon juice
1 1/2   cups halved green grapes
1   Tbsp cornstarch or arrowroot powder
2   Tbsp water

Exchanges
1 Carbohydrate
4 Very Lean Meat
Calories 234
Calories from Fat 48
Total Fat.................... 5 g
Saturated Fat .... 1 g
Cholesterol .... 73 mg
Sodium................. 112 mg
Total Carbohydrate 18 g
Dietary Fiber........... 1 g
Sugars .... 9 g
Protein .... 28 g

1. In a plastic zip-top bag, combine the chicken breasts with the flour, pepper, and salt. Shake well.

2. In a large skillet over medium-high heat, heat the oil. Add the chicken breasts and sauté on each side for 5 minutes. Remove the chicken from the skillet.

3. In the same skillet, sauté the onion in the remaining pan drippings. Add the chicken broth and orange marmalade. Stir well. Add the rosemary and lemon juice and cook for 3 minutes. Add the grapes and cook for 5 minutes. Add the chicken back to the skillet and cook for 10 more minutes.

4. In a small measuring cup, combine the cornstarch or arrowroot powder with the water. Add to the skillet and cook until sauce is thickened. Add ground pepper to taste.

Perfect Poultry

95

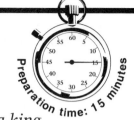

Bombay Chicken

Total Servings: 6
Serving Size: 3–4 oz

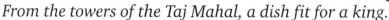

From the towers of the Taj Mahal, a dish fit for a king.

2 tsp corn oil	
1 medium onion, minced	
2 garlic cloves, minced	
1 1/2 lb chicken breasts, boned, skinned, halved, and cut into 2-inch pieces	
1 Tbsp curry powder	
1 cup diagonally sliced carrots	
1 cup cauliflower florets	
1 1/2 cups evaporated nonfat milk	
1/2 cup canned chickpeas, drained	
1/4 cup raisins	
1/2 cup frozen peas, thawed and drained	
1 Tbsp cornstarch or arrowroot powder	
2 Tbsp water	

Exchanges
1 1/2 Carbohydrate
1 Vegetable
4 Very Lean Meat

Calories	280
Calories from Fat	48
Total Fat	5 g
Saturated Fat	1 g
Cholesterol	71 mg
Sodium	185 mg
Total Carbohydrate	25 g
Dietary Fiber	3 g
Sugars	14 g
Protein	33 g

1. Heat the oil in a large saucepot over medium-high heat. Add the onion, garlic, and chicken and sauté until the chicken is almost cooked through, about 5 minutes. Add the curry powder and cook for 3 more minutes.

2. Place the carrots and cauliflower together on a steamer and steam over boiling water for 5–6 minutes. Remove from the heat and add to the chicken. Add the evaporated milk and cook for 5 minutes over medium heat.

3. Add the chickpeas, raisins, and peas. Mix together the cornstarch or arrowroot powder with the water. Add to the chicken mixture. Cook until sauce is thickened, about 3–5 minutes.

Chicken Paprikash

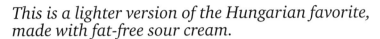

Total Servings: 6
Serving Size: 3–4 oz

Preparation time: 10 minutes

This is a lighter version of the Hungarian favorite,
made with fat-free sour cream.

2 tsp canola oil	
1 medium onion, diced	
3 whole chicken breasts (8 oz each, 1 1/2 lb total), halved, boned, and skinned	
2 Tbsp paprika	
1/2 cup low-fat, reduced-sodium chicken broth	
1 cup fat-free sour cream	
Fresh ground pepper and salt to taste	

Exchanges
1/2 Carbohydrate
4 Very Lean Meat
1/2 Fat

Calories	198
Calories from Fat	43
Total Fat	5 g
Saturated Fat	0.9 g
Cholesterol	71 mg
Sodium	151 mg
Total Carbohydrate	10 g
Dietary Fiber	1 g
Sugars	5 g
Protein	27 g

1. In a skillet over medium-high heat, heat the oil. Add the onion and sauté for 5 minutes.

2. In a plastic zip-top bag, shake the chicken breasts with 1 Tbsp of the paprika. Cook the chicken on each side until browned, about 5 minutes. Add the chicken broth to the skillet, bring to a boil, lower the heat, and cover for 10 minutes.

3. When broth has evaporated, remove the chicken from the skillet. Add the sour cream, remaining paprika, pepper, and salt. Heat over low heat for 2 minutes. Add the chicken breasts. Serve over hot noodles, if desired (not included in nutrient analysis).

Chicken Marsala

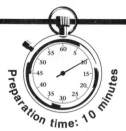

Total Servings: 6
Serving Size: 3–4 oz

Every cook needs a good Italian chicken marsala recipe.

2 tsp olive oil
1 medium onion, chopped
1 1/2 lb whole chicken breasts, halved, boned, and skinned, pounded until 1/4 inch thick
1 cup dry marsala wine
1 Tbsp cornstarch or arrowroot powder
3/4 cup low-fat, reduced-sodium chicken broth
Fresh ground pepper and salt to taste

Exchanges	
1/2 Carbohydrate	
4 Very Lean Meat	
Calories	182
Calories from Fat	43
Total Fat	5 g
Saturated Fat	1 g
Cholesterol	69 mg
Sodium	99 mg
Total Carbohydrate	4 g
Dietary Fiber	0 g
Sugars	2 g
Protein	26 g

1. In a large skillet over medium-high heat, heat the oil. Add the onion and sauté for 5 minutes. Add the chicken and cook on each side for 5 minutes.

2. Add the wine and cook for about 4 minutes until the wine looks syrupy.

3. In a small cup, dissolve the cornstarch or arrowroot powder in the broth. Add to the chicken and cook until the sauce is thickened, about 2 minutes. Add pepper and salt to taste.

Turkey Burritos

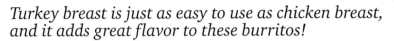

Total Servings: 6
Serving Size: 3–4 oz in one 6-inch tortilla

Turkey breast is just as easy to use as chicken breast,
and it adds great flavor to these burritos!

      2 tsp olive oil
      1 medium onion, chopped
      2 garlic cloves, minced
  1/2 cup diced green peppers
      1 Tbsp chili powder
1 1/2 lb lean ground turkey breast
      1 cup diced tomatoes
  1/2 cup corn kernels
      6 6-inch tortillas, heated (To heat: wrap
          in foil and place in a 300°F oven
          until warm and soft or wrap three
          tortillas in two damp paper towels
          and microwave on high for 1 minute.)
      1 cup salsa

Exchanges	
1 1/2 Starch	
1 Vegetable	
4 Very Lean Meat	
Calories	274
Calories from Fat	41
Total Fat	5 g
Saturated Fat	1 g
Cholesterol	75 mg
Sodium	367 mg
Total Carbohydrate	26 g
Dietary Fiber	3 g
Sugars	6 g
Protein	32 g

1. In a skillet over medium-high heat, heat the oil. Add the onion and garlic and sauté for 5 minutes. Add the peppers and sauté for 3 more minutes.

2. Add the chili powder and ground turkey and sauté until the turkey is no longer pink. Add the tomatoes and corn and cook 2 more minutes.

3. Spoon some of the turkey mixture into each warm tortilla. Roll up. Serve each tortilla with 2 Tbsp of salsa.

Grilled Turkey with Garlic Sauce

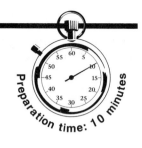

Total Servings: 6
Serving Size: 3–4 oz with 2–3 Tbsp sauce

You can also use this sauce to top chicken.

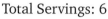

1/3 cup minced parsley
5 garlic cloves, minced
1/3 cup lemon juice
3 Tbsp olive oil
1 tsp paprika
1 tsp cumin
Dash cayenne pepper
1 1/2 lb turkey breast slices, pounded until
1/4 inch thick
1 Tbsp olive oil for brushing on turkey
while grilling

Exchanges	
4 Lean Meat	
Calories	210
Calories from Fat	89
Total Fat	10 g
Saturated Fat	1.4 g
Cholesterol	74 mg
Sodium	53 mg
Total Carbohydrate	2 g
Dietary Fiber	0 g
Sugars	1 g
Protein	27 g

1. In a blender, blend all sauce ingredients together.

2. Grill or broil the turkey breasts 6 inches from the heat source, brushing with olive oil to keep moist. Grill on each side about 4 minutes.

3. Top each slice with some of the sauce (about 2–3 Tbsp per slice).

Diabetic Meals in 30 Minutes—Or Less!

Turkey Provençal

Total Servings: 6
Serving Size: 3–4 oz

The delicious smell of this dish will draw an audience to your kitchen!

Preparation time: 15 minutes

1 1/2 lb turkey fillets
   2 Tbsp unbleached white flour
     Fresh ground pepper and salt to taste
   2 tsp olive oil
   1 medium onion, diced
   2 garlic cloves, minced
1 1/2 cups crushed canned tomatoes
   1 Tbsp fresh chopped thyme
 1/4 cup sliced black olives
   2 tsp capers
 1/2 cup minced parsley

Exchanges	
2 Vegetable	
4 Very Lean Meat	
Calories	189
Calories from Fat	27
Total Fat	3 g
Saturated Fat	1 g
Cholesterol	75 mg
Sodium	294 mg
Total Carbohydrate	10 g
Dietary Fiber	2 g
Sugars	5 g
Protein	29 g

1. In a plastic zip-top bag, place the turkey fillets with the flour, pepper, and salt. Shake the bag until the turkey fillets are coated with flour.

2. In a large skillet over medium heat, heat the oil. Add the turkey fillets and sauté on each side for 4 minutes. Remove from the skillet.

3. In the same skillet, sauté the onion and garlic for 5 minutes until the onions begin to brown. Add the crushed tomatoes. Bring to a boil. Lower the heat and let simmer for 5 minutes.

4. Add the turkey, thyme, olives, and capers to the skillet. Simmer over low heat for 10 minutes. Add the parsley and serve.

Stuffed Zucchini Boats

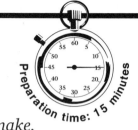

Total Servings: 6
Serving Size: 3–4 oz

This dish is almost as much fun to eat as it is to make.

3 medium zucchini
1 1/2 lb lean ground turkey breast
1 small onion, minced
1/2 cup finely diced carrot
1/2 cup finely diced red pepper
2 tsp fresh minced basil
1 tsp fresh minced oregano
1 egg, beaten
1 cup store-bought, reduced-fat, low-sugar spaghetti sauce

Exchanges		
2 Vegetable		
4 Very Lean Meat		
Calories		171
Calories from Fat		7
Total Fat		1 g
Saturated Fat		0 g
Cholesterol		110 mg
Sodium		207 mg
Total Carbohydrate		10 g
Dietary Fiber		2 g
Sugars		6 g
Protein		30 g

1. Cut each zucchini in half lengthwise and scoop out the inside of each zucchini, leaving a 1-inch shell. Then cut the zucchini boat in half crosswise to make six boats. Mince the scooped-out zucchini.

2. Place the hollowed-out zucchini boats in a saucepan and cover with water. Bring water to a boil and boil the boats for 5 minutes. Drain and set aside.

3. In a large skillet, sauté the ground turkey until cooked through, about 6 minutes. Remove the turkey from the skillet. Add the onion to the pan drippings and sauté for 5 minutes. Add the carrot, red pepper, and reserved minced zucchini. Add the basil and oregano. Add in the ground turkey and egg and mix well.

4. Fill each zucchini boat with the turkey mixture. Place the zucchini boats in a preheated oven at 350°F and bake uncovered for 10 minutes. Serve with heated spaghetti sauce drizzled on each zucchini boat (about 2 Tbsp per person).

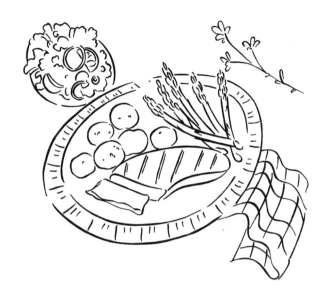

LEAN BEEF AND PORK

Although it is wise to limit your consumption of high-fat beef, pork, and other cuts of meat, you can still include lean cuts in a wholesome meal plan. Lean beef is still a wonderful source of protein, zinc, iron, and vitamin B. Also, pork is leaner than it used to be, thanks to new farm feeding techniques. Try to use the pork tenderloin portion. Just remember to trim the fat carefully off all cuts of meat and include vegetables and salads with your meal.

FRENCH BURGERS

MEXICAN BEEF STIR-FRY

WARM ASIAN BEEF SALAD

FIESTA FAJITAS

GRILLED SIRLOIN WITH CAPER MUSTARD SAUCE

SOUTH SEA ISLAND PORK KABOBS

PORK TENDERLOIN WITH COUNTRY MUSTARD CREAM SAUCE

PORK OLÉ SALAD WITH ROASTED PUMPKIN SEED DRESSING

GOOD OL' PORK BARBECUE

French Burgers

Total Servings: 6
Serving Size: 3–4 oz

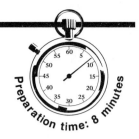

Imagine savoring this juicy burger by the Eiffel Tower!

1 1/2 lb lean ground beef (95% lean, 5% fat)
3 Tbsp Dijon mustard
1 Tbsp minced thyme
1 Tbsp white wine
2 Tbsp minced onion
2 garlic cloves, minced

Exchanges	
3 Lean Meat	
Calories	171
Calories from Fat	59
Total Fat	7 g
Saturated Fat	2.9 g
Cholesterol	73 mg
Sodium	250 mg
Total Carbohydrate	2 g
Dietary Fiber	0 g
Sugars	1 g
Protein	24 g

Combine all ingredients. Shape into six patties. Broil until done as desired (3–4 minutes for rare, 5–7 minutes for medium, and 8–9 minutes for well done).

Mexican Beef Stir-Fry

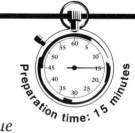

Total Servings: 6
Serving Size: 3–4 oz

Although this dish is made in a wok, it has a true Southwest flavor.

1	Tbsp canola oil
1 1/2	lb lean sirloin steak, cut into 3-inch strips, trimmed of all fat
3	garlic cloves, minced
1	medium onion, minced
1	small red pepper, cut into thin strips
2	tsp chili powder
2	Tbsp lime juice
1	tsp cumin

Exchanges

1 Vegetable
3 Lean Meat

Calories	180
Calories from Fat	67
Total Fat	7 g
Saturated Fat	2 g
Cholesterol	65 mg
Sodium	58 mg
Total Carbohydrate	4 g
Dietary Fiber	1 g
Sugars	3 g
Protein	23 g

1. In a wok over medium-high heat, heat the oil. Add the beef and sauté until the beef loses its pinkness. Drain any accumulated fat. Remove the beef from the wok.

2. Add the garlic and onions and sauté for 5 minutes. Add the red pepper and sauté for 5 more minutes.

3. Add the chili powder and lime juice to coat the vegetables. Add the beef back to the skillet and add the cumin. Heat 1 more minute.

Diabetic Meals in 30 Minutes—Or Less!

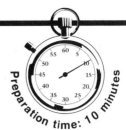

Warm Asian Beef Salad

Total Servings: 6
Serving Size: 3–4 oz

Preparation time: 10 minutes

When the cold weather comes, you can still eat a hearty, healthy salad.

Beef
      1 Tbsp peanut oil
1 1/2 lb lean flank steak, cut into
             3-inch strips
      2 garlic cloves, minced

Dressing
  1/2 cup rice vinegar
      1 Tbsp oyster sauce
      1 Tbsp lite soy sauce
      1 tsp honey

Salad greens
      6 cups torn romaine lettuce
  1/2 cup sliced celery
  1/2 cup sliced scallions

Garnish
      1 Tbsp sesame seeds

Exchanges	
1 Vegetable	
3 Lean Meat	
Calories	199
Calories from Fat	82
Total Fat	9 g
Saturated Fat	3 g
Cholesterol	39 mg
Sodium	222 mg
Total Carbohydrate	5 g
Dietary Fiber	2 g
Sugars	2 g
Protein	24 g

1. In a wok over medium-high heat, heat the oil. Add the steak and stir-fry until the steak loses its pinkness. Add the garlic and stir-fry 1 more minute.

2. In a small cup, combine the dressing ingredients. Add to the steak and bring to a boil. Remove the wok from the stove.

3. Combine all the salad ingredients. Place the warm steak mixture on top. Garnish with sesame seeds and serve.

Lean Beef and Pork

Fiesta Fajitas

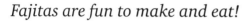
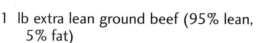

Total Servings: 6
Serving Size: about 2 oz beef and 1/4 cup vegetables
in one 6-inch flour tortilla

Fajitas are fun to make and eat!

1	lb extra lean ground beef (95% lean, 5% fat)
1	medium onion, diced
2	garlic cloves, minced
1/4	cup each diced red and green pepper
1/2	cup corn kernels (fresh or frozen)
1/2	cup diced tomato
3	tsp chili powder
1	tsp cumin
6	6-inch flour tortillas, heated (To heat: wrap in foil and place in a 300°F oven until warm and soft or wrap 3 tortillas in two damp paper towels and microwave on high for 1 minute.)
1	cup salsa (about 2 Tbsp per serving)

Exchanges

1 1/2 Starch

1 Vegetable

2 Lean Meat

Calories	245
Calories from Fat	63
Total Fat	7 g
Saturated Fat	2.5 g
Cholesterol	49 mg
Sodium	513 mg
Total Carbohydrate	26 g
Dietary Fiber	3 g
Sugars	4 g
Protein	20 g

1. In a large skillet over medium-high heat, sauté the ground beef until cooked through, about 8 minutes. Drain from skillet, leaving 3 tsp of pan drippings. Set beef aside.

2. In the same skillet, sauté the onion, garlic, and peppers for 10 minutes. Add the corn and tomato and cook for 5 more minutes. Add the chili powder, the cumin, and the beef and cook for 1 more minute.

3. Spoon some of the fajita mixture into each warm tortilla. Roll up. Serve each tortilla with 2 Tbsp of salsa.

Grilled Sirloin with Caper Mustard Sauce

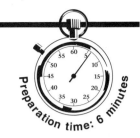

Total Servings: 6
Serving Size: 3–4 oz sirloin with 1–2 Tbsp sauce

This is a delicious main dish with a creamy, mustard-flavored sauce.

Beef
1 1/2 lb lean sirloin
1 Tbsp coarsely crushed black peppercorns

Sauce
1/2 cup reduced-fat mayonnaise
1/4 cup Dijon mustard
1 Tbsp small capers
Fresh ground pepper and salt to taste

Exchanges	
1/2 Carbohydrate	
3 Very Lean Meat	
1/2 Fat	
Calories	181
Calories from Fat	60
Total Fat	7 g
Saturated Fat	2 g
Cholesterol	65 mg
Sodium	384 mg
Total Carbohydrate	6 g
Dietary Fiber	0 g
Sugars	5 g
Protein	23 g

1. With the heel of your hand, press the peppercorns into the top side of the steak. Grill the sirloin 6 inches from the heat source until done as desired (about 12–13 minutes for rare, 15–16 minutes for medium, and 18 minutes for well done). Slice into thin slices.

2. Combine all sauce ingredients. Serve the steak with the mustard sauce.

South Sea Island Pork Kabobs

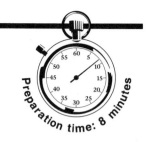

Total Servings: 6
Serving Size: 3–4 oz

Ginger and pineapple juice concentrate give this dish a strong fruit flavor.

Pork
1 1/2 lb lean pork tenderloin, cut into 2- to
     3-inch cubes

Marinade
2 Tbsp pineapple juice concentrate
1 Tbsp minced ginger
1/3 cup water
2 Tbsp lime juice
2 tsp dark rum

Exchanges		
4 Very Lean Meat		
Calories 149		
Calories from Fat 37		
Total Fat..................... 4 g		
Saturated Fat .... 1 g		
Cholesterol .... 66 mg		
Sodium.................... 48 mg		
Total Carbohydrate . 2 g		
Dietary Fiber............ 0 g		
Sugars .... 2 g		
Protein...................... 24 g		

1. Place the pork cubes in a plastic zip-top bag.

2. Combine all of the marinade ingredients. Add to the pork. Let the pork marinate for several hours.

3. Thread six 8- to 10-inch skewers with the marinated pork. Grill 6 inches from the heat source for about 10–15 minutes, rotating the skewers. Make sure the pork is completely cooked through (there should be no traces of pink). Serve over rice if desired.

Pork Tenderloin with Country Mustard Cream Sauce

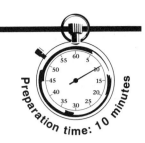

Preparation time: 10 minutes

Total Servings: 6
Serving Size: 3–4 oz pork with 1/4 cup sauce

Try to use coarse Dijon mustard for a special country taste.

2 tsp olive oil	
1 1/2 lb pork tenderloin, cut into 3- to 4-oz fillets	
1 cup diced onion	
1 12-oz can evaporated nonfat milk	
2 Tbsp coarse Dijon mustard	
2 tsp fresh chopped rosemary	
2 tsp minced chives	
1/4 cup minced parsley	
Fresh ground pepper to taste	

Exchanges

1/2 Starch
4 Very Lean Meat
1/2 Fat

Calories	212
Calories from Fat	54
Total Fat	6 g
Saturated Fat	2 g
Cholesterol	68 mg
Sodium	177 mg
Total Carbohydrate	10 g
Dietary Fiber	1 g
Sugars	7 g
Protein	28 g

1. In a large skillet over medium heat, heat the olive oil. Add the pork slices and sauté on each side for 6–7 minutes until no pink remains. Remove the pork from the skillet.

2. In the pan drippings, sauté the onion for 10 minutes. Add the evaporated milk, mustard, and rosemary. Bring to a boil, then lower the heat to simmer. Add the pork and simmer for 5 minutes. Add the chives and parsley. Grind in the pepper and simmer for 3 more minutes.

Pork Olé Salad with Roasted Pumpkin Seed Dressing

Total Servings: 6
Serving Size: 3–4 oz pork and 1/4 cup vegetables

Just add crusty bread to this satisfying summer salad. Since it is sometimes hard to find pumpkin seeds sold in small quantities, buy a larger batch and freeze the remainder to keep it fresh.

Salad

1 1/2	lb cooked pork tenderloin, sliced into 3-inch strips
1/2	cup cooked yellow corn kernels
1	cup diced red pepper
1/2	cup diced red onion
1/2	cup diced jicama (if you can't find jicama, you can omit it)
1/2	cup diced tomato
1/4	cup diced mango or papaya

Dressing

2	Tbsp raw, unsalted pumpkin seeds
6	Tbsp fresh lime juice
2	Tbsp fresh orange juice
2	tsp olive oil
2	Tbsp fat-free sour cream
2	tsp minced cilantro
1	tsp chili powder

Butter lettuce leaves

Exchanges	
1/2 Carbohydrate	
1 Vegetable	
3 Lean Meat	
Calories	221
Calories from Fat	71
Total Fat	8 g
Saturated Fat	2 g
Cholesterol	66 mg
Sodium	64 mg
Total Carbohydrate	11 g
Dietary Fiber	2 g
Sugars	4 g
Protein	27 g

1. In a large salad bowl, combine all of the salad ingredients.

2. Place the pumpkin seeds in a small dry skillet over medium heat. Toast the seeds until they lightly brown. Remove from the heat.

3. In a blender or food processor, combine the seeds with the juices and oil. Blend for 30 seconds. By hand, fold in the sour cream, cilantro, and chili powder. Toss the dressing with the salad and serve on butter lettuce.

Good Ol' Pork Barbecue

Total Servings: 6
Serving Size: 3–4 oz with 1–2 oz bread

This recipe is high in sodium due to the catsup. If you need to reduce sodium in your diet, try using reduced-sodium catsup.

2 Tbsp canola oil	
1 small onion, minced	
1 cup catsup	
2 Tbsp red wine vinegar	
1 Tbsp honey	
2 Tbsp Worcestershire sauce	
1 cup water	
2 tsp paprika	
2 tsp chili powder	
1/2 tsp cayenne	
1 1/2 lb cooked pork tenderloin, shredded or cubed into small pieces	
6 slices toasted French, Italian, or multigrain bread	

Exchanges

2 Carbohydrate

3 Lean Meat

Calories	320
Calories from Fat	94
Total Fat	10 g
Saturated Fat	2 g
Cholesterol	66 mg
Sodium	730 mg
Total Carbohydrate	31 g
Dietary Fiber	3 g
Sugars	10 g
Protein	27 g

1. To make the sauce, combine all ingredients except the pork and bread in a saucepan. Simmer uncovered over medium heat for 15 minutes, until the onion has softened.

2. Prepare the pork and add it to the sauce. Continue to simmer for 5 minutes.

3. Pile the pork filling evenly over each bread slice. Eat with a fork.

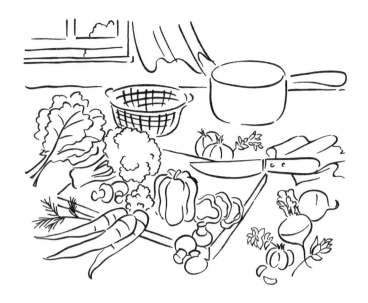

Very Quick Vegetables

The phrase "strive for five" is really true when it comes to eating vegetables. Unfortunately, most of the time vegetables just end up as lifeless blobs on our plates. This chapter provides fast, delicious vegetable recipes that everyone will enjoy. You can use either fresh or frozen vegetables, but avoid canned varieties because of the high sodium content and dull flavor.

Although eating fresh vegetables is a tasty part of your healthy lifestyle, avoid the tendency to overbuy them. For the freshest flavor, try to store vegetables for no more than 2 days in your refrigerator. If you want them to last longer, your best bet would be to buy frozen veggies. The new vegetable plastic bags available, with tiny holes to help the vegetables breathe, will keep your vegetables fresher. Look for this in the plastic bag and foil aisle of your grocery store.

For the best nutritional value, try to stick with the vegetable "powerhouses," such as broccoli, cauliflower, carrots, peppers (particularly the red ones), beets, and all of the greens, such as mustard, kale, chard, collards, and spinach.

VEGETABLE COOKING METHODS

CARROTS WITH ORANGE GLAZE

GARDEN-FRESH GREEN BEANS AND TOMATOES WITH OREGANO

ASPARAGUS IN BROWN SAUCE

TRIPLE CABBAGE DELIGHT

SESAME KALE

FRESH SPINACH AND MUSHROOM MEDLEY

SNOW PEAS WITH WATER CHESTNUTS AND BAMBOO SHOOTS

BABY RED POTATOES WITH FRESH HERBS

GRILLED SUMMER SQUASH AND ZUCCHINI

SAUCY GREEN BEANS AND CAULIFLOWER

Vegetable Cooking Methods

Many different techniques are available to cook vegetables. Use methods like the ones below to keep vegetables crisp, colorful, and full of nutrients.

Steaming: This technique requires a little more time than boiling, but preserves levels of some nutrients like vitamin C, which are diminished by boiling. Steaming helps retain delicate vegetable flavors and is therefore better suited to mild-tasting vegetables, such as summer squash, carrots, and beets, rather than strong-tasting vegetables, such as Brussels sprouts and cabbage. For proper steaming, place vegetables on a steamer rack above boiling water in a saucepan. Cover the saucepan tightly to keep in the steam. Replenish the water if you need to during the steaming process. Pasta pots often come with steamer inserts, or use Chinese bamboo steamers that stack and enable you to steam many items at once. Folding steamers fit in most pots.

Stir-frying: This is a very quick method of preparing vegetables. Keep the heat relatively high, and continuously toss the cut vegetables over the heat until they are done, but are still slightly crisp. A wok is the best vehicle for stir-frying, but a heavy skillet will do. Make sure your pan is hot enough or the food will absorb too much oil and stick to the sides.

Grilling: This method is suitable for certain vegetables. Sweet peppers, tomatoes, large mushrooms, potatoes, sweet potatoes, and corn are all delicious when grilled. Simply brush the vegetables with a little oil to prevent drying. You can place small pieces of vegetables in foil and then set them on the grill. The rack should be about 6 inches from the heat source, and the heat should be about medium.

Microwaving: This technique is best for vegetables you need done in a hurry that would normally take a long time to cook. Usually, vegetables should be microwaved at high power.

Roasting: This is a favorite method of cooking winter squash, potatoes, sweet potatoes, eggplant, peppers, and tomatoes. The dry heat preserves the flavor of these veggies better than steaming. Moisten the vegetable with oil or a marinade and bake in the oven until tender. You can also scatter these vegetables around a chicken or roast to absorb the meat juices as they cook.

Braising: This method cooks vegetables slowly with a small amount of liquid, which you can then use to make a sauce. For added flavor, the braising liquid should be either soup stock or water enhanced with onions, garlic, or herbs. The best braising pan is a deep sauté pan with a lid; a heavy, wide casserole; or a Dutch oven. Braising is best for slow-cooking vegetables, such as large pieces of carrot, potatoes, or eggplant.

Use Herbs and Spices: Try experimenting with different herbs and spices. Reaching for the salt shaker all the time limits your culinary imagination (and adds unwanted sodium to your meal plan). Vegetables have a nice, sweet flavor when cooked properly, so a sprinkle or two of salt is all you really need.

When you just feel like tossing in some herbs for flavor, here are some good matches. Fresh herbs will taste the best. You can use dried herbs, but for best flavor results, make sure they are not more than a year old.

- Tarragon for asparagus
- Basil for tomatoes, carrots, and potatoes
- Thyme for carrots and summer squash
- Rosemary for potatoes, peas, and spinach
- Mint for peas
- Dill for broccoli, corn, and beets
- Marjoram for broccoli

Use about 1 Tbsp of chopped herbs for 2 cups of vegetables. Just take a pair of scissors and snip the herb right into the cooked vegetable. Add fresh ground pepper, a dash of olive oil, and serve!

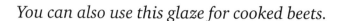

Carrots with Orange Glaze

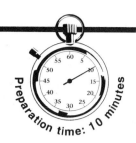

Preparation time: 10 minutes

Total Servings: 6
Serving Size: 1/2 cup

You can also use this glaze for cooked beets.

Carrots
    3 cups diagonally sliced, peeled carrots

Glaze
  1/3 cup fresh orange juice
  1/4 cup water
    1 Tbsp fresh lemon juice
    1 Tbsp honey
    1 tsp cinnamon
  1/2 tsp nutmeg
    1 Tbsp cornstarch or arrowroot
    2 Tbsp water

Garnish
    Fresh mint leaves

Exchanges	
2 Vegetable	
Calories	54
Calories from Fat	1
Total Fat	0 g
Saturated Fat	0 g
Cholesterol	0 mg
Sodium	48 mg
Total Carbohydrate	13 g
Dietary Fiber	2 g
Sugars	7 g
Protein	1 g

1. Prepare the carrots by steaming them over boiling water on a steamer rack, covered, for 5 minutes. Drain and set aside.

2. In a small saucepan over medium heat, combine the orange juice, water, lemon juice, honey, and spices. Bring to a boil. Reduce the heat and cook for 3 minutes.

3. Combine the cornstarch or arrowroot with the water. Add to the orange juice mixture and cook over low heat until thickened. Pour the orange glaze over the carrots and serve. Garnish with mint leaves.

Garden-Fresh Green Beans and Tomatoes with Oregano

Total Servings: 6
Serving Size: 1/2 cup

Preparation time: 8 minutes

Try to purchase vine-ripened tomatoes for this straight-from-the-field side dish.

2 tsp olive oil
1/4 cup diced onion
2 garlic cloves, minced
2 cups cut green beans (trim ends and cut green beans in 1-inch lengths)
1/4 cup low-fat, reduced-sodium chicken broth
1 medium tomato, diced
1 Tbsp fresh minced oregano
1 Tbsp minced parsley
Fresh ground pepper and salt to taste

Exchanges	
1 Vegetable	
1/2 Fat	
Calories	39
Calories from Fat	17
Total Fat	2 g
Saturated Fat	0 g
Cholesterol	0 mg
Sodium	32 mg
Total Carbohydrate	6 g
Dietary Fiber	2 g
Sugars	2 g
Protein	1 g

1. In a wok or heavy skillet over medium-high heat, heat the oil. Add the onion and garlic and sauté for 3 minutes (do not let the garlic brown). Add the green beans and broth, cover, and steam for 3 minutes.

2. Add the diced tomato, cover, and steam 30 seconds. Add the oregano, parsley, pepper, and salt and steam for 30 seconds more. Serve.

Asparagus in Brown Sauce

Total Servings: 6
Serving Size: 1/2 cup

Preparation time: 8 minutes

To prepare asparagus, break off the bottom end and diagonally slice it into 1-inch lengths. Choose asparagus that has tightly closed buds and stems that are neither too thin nor too thick. Asparagus is best in the spring.

Asparagus
- 2 tsp peanut oil
- 3 garlic cloves, minced
- 6 cups sliced asparagus (about 2 lb)

Sauce
- 1/2 cup low-fat, reduced-sodium chicken broth
- 2 Tbsp lite soy sauce
- 2 Tbsp rice vinegar
- 1 Tbsp oyster sauce
- 1 tsp Tabasco® sauce
- 1 tsp sesame oil
- 1 1/2 Tbsp cornstarch or arrowroot powder
- 3 Tbsp water

Garnish
- 1/4 cup minced scallions

Exchanges	
2 Vegetable	
1/2 Fat	
Calories	80
Calories from Fat	27
Total Fat	3 g
Saturated Fat	1 g
Cholesterol	0 mg
Sodium	340 mg
Total Carbohydrate	11 g
Dietary Fiber	4 g
Sugars	5 g
Protein	5 g

1. In a wok over medium-high heat, heat the oil. Add the garlic and sauté for 20 seconds. Add the asparagus and stir-fry for 3 minutes.

2. Combine all the sauce ingredients, except the cornstarch or arrowroot powder and the water. Add to the asparagus, cover, and steam for 1 minute.

3. Add the cornstarch or arrowroot powder to the water and stir until it is completely dissolved. Add this mixture to the sauce. Cook until sauce is thickened, about 1 minute. Garnish with scallions.

Very Quick Vegetables

Triple Cabbage Delight

Total Servings: 6
Serving Size: 1/2 cup

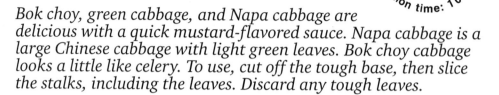

Bok choy, green cabbage, and Napa cabbage are delicious with a quick mustard-flavored sauce. Napa cabbage is a large Chinese cabbage with light green leaves. Bok choy cabbage looks a little like celery. To use, cut off the tough base, then slice the stalks, including the leaves. Discard any tough leaves.

Cabbage

1 cup sliced bok choy cabbage
1 cup sliced green cabbage (1/4 small head)
1 cup sliced Napa cabbage

Sauce

1/2 cup Dijon mustard
3 Tbsp lite soy sauce
1 tsp sugar
2 Tbsp rice vinegar

Exchanges	
1 Vegetable	
Calories	30
Calories from Fat	8
Total Fat	1 g
Saturated Fat	0 g
Cholesterol	0 mg
Sodium	559 mg
Total Carbohydrate	4 g
Dietary Fiber	1 g
Sugars	4 g
Protein	1 g

1. In a large pot of boiling water, add the sliced cabbages and cook for just 1 minute. Drain and splash the cabbage with cold water.

2. Mix all ingredients for the sauce. Add the mustard sauce to the cabbage and toss well. Serve chilled. This dish is good with a fish entree.

Sesame Kale

Total Servings: 6
Serving Size: 1/2 cup

Kale deserves a wider audience in this country. This vitamin- and fiber-packed vegetable is so easy to prepare.

Preparation time: 8 minutes

1 1/2 lb kale
   2 tsp sesame oil
   2 garlic cloves, minced
1/4 cup low-fat, reduced-sodium chicken
      broth
   1 Tbsp lite soy sauce
   2 tsp toasted sesame seeds
      Fresh ground pepper to taste

Exchanges	
1 Vegetable	
1/2 Fat	
Calories	52
Calories from Fat	23
Total Fat	3 g
Saturated Fat	0 g
Cholesterol	0 mg
Sodium	127 mg
Total Carbohydrate	6 g
Dietary Fiber	2 g
Sugars	3 g
Protein	2 g

1. Wash the kale, but let the water cling to it. Cut off and discard the tough stems. Slice the leaves once down the middle, then cut them crosswise into 1-inch-wide strips.

2. In a wok, heat the oil. Add the garlic. Sauté for 10 seconds. Add the kale and the broth. Cover and steam for 3 minutes until the kale wilts. Add the soy sauce.

3. Top the kale with sesame seeds and fresh ground pepper. Serve.

Fresh Spinach and Mushroom Medley

Total Servings: 6
Serving Size: 1/2 cup

Preparation time: 5 minutes

Popeye was right when he dug into his spinach! Rich in nutrients with a slight peppery flavor, fresh spinach can't be beat.

2 tsp olive oil
2 garlic cloves, minced
1/2 cup canned straw mushrooms, drained (Look in the Asian food section of your grocery store or substitute regular mushrooms.)
3/4 lb fresh spinach leaves, washed (do not dry!), stemmed, and coarsely chopped (about 2 1/2 cups)
2 Tbsp fresh lemon juice
Fresh ground pepper and salt to taste

Exchanges	
1 Vegetable	
Calories	34
Calories from Fat	15
Total Fat	2 g
Saturated Fat	0 g
Cholesterol	0 mg
Sodium	126 mg
Total Carbohydrate	4 g
Dietary Fiber	2 g
Sugars	1 g
Protein	2 g

1. In a wok or heavy skillet over medium-high heat, heat the oil. Add the garlic and sauté for 10 seconds. Add the mushrooms and sauté for 2 minutes.

2. Add the spinach, cover, and steam for 2–3 minutes until it wilts. Add the lemon juice and pepper and serve.

Snow Peas with Water Chestnuts and Bamboo Shoots

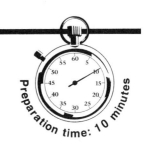

Preparation time: 10 minutes

Total Servings: 6
Serving Size: 1/2 cup

Snow peas are one of the quickest-cooking vegetables. Be sure to buy only fresh snow peas—anything else pales in comparison!

2	tsp peanut oil
1/2	cup diced onion
1/4	cup diced celery
2	cups trimmed fresh snow peas
1/2	cup sliced water chestnuts
1/2	cup sliced bamboo shoots
1/2	cup low-fat, reduced-sodium chicken broth
	Fresh ground pepper and salt to taste

Exchanges

1 Vegetable
1/2 Fat

Calories	51
Calories from Fat	17
Total Fat	2 g
Saturated Fat	0 g
Cholesterol	0 mg
Sodium	41 mg
Total Carbohydrate	7 g
Dietary Fiber	2 g
Sugars	4 g
Protein	2 g

1. In a wok over medium-high heat, heat the oil. Add the onion and celery and stir-fry for 3 minutes.

2. Add the snow peas, water chestnuts, bamboo shoots, and broth. Cover and steam 1–2 minutes.

3. Add the pepper and salt to taste. Snow peas should still be crisp and bright green when served.

Baby Red Potatoes with Fresh Herbs

Preparation time: 10 minutes

Total Servings: 6
Serving Size: 1/2 cup

When choosing potatoes for this recipe, seek out very small ones. They will be sweet and moist, and it only takes about 10 minutes for them to boil.

3 cups (about 1 1/2 lb) baby red potatoes, washed and scrubbed (do not peel)
1 Tbsp olive oil
4 garlic cloves, minced
2 tsp minced dill
2 tsp minced rosemary
1 tsp minced mint
1 tsp minced rosemary
Fresh ground pepper to taste

Exchanges	
1 1/2 Starch	
Calories	121
Calories from Fat	22
Total Fat	2 g
Saturated Fat	0 g
Cholesterol	0 mg
Sodium	7 mg
Total Carbohydrate	23 g
Dietary Fiber	2 g
Sugars	3 g
Protein	2 g

1. In a medium saucepan, cover the potatoes with water and boil for about 10 minutes. Drain and place in a bowl.
2. Toss the potatoes with the remaining ingredients and serve.

Grilled Summer Squash and Zucchini

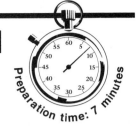

Preparation time: 7 minutes

Total Servings: 6
Serving Size: 1/2 small zucchini or squash

Grilling yellow squash and zucchini really brings out their flavors.

Squash

    3 small summer squash (combination of zucchini and yellow)

Basting sauce

    1 garlic clove, minced
  1/2 tsp paprika
  1/2 tsp cumin
    2 Tbsp olive oil
    1 Tbsp fresh lemon juice

Exchanges	
1 Vegetable	
1/2 Fat	
Calories	29
Calories from Fat	21
Total Fat	2 g
Saturated Fat	0 g
Cholesterol	0 mg
Sodium	1 mg
Total Carbohydrate	2 g
Dietary Fiber	1 g
Sugars	1 g
Protein	0 g

1. Halve each squash, but do not peel. Combine all ingredients for sauce.

2. To grill, place the squash on a rack over medium-hot coals with the rack set 6 inches from the heat source. Baste with some of the sauce. Grill the squash about 5 minutes on each side, basting frequently with sauce. Serve.

Saucy Green Beans and Cauliflower

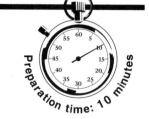

Total Servings: 6
Serving Size: 1/2 cup

Just a touch of sharp bleu cheese makes this dish special!

Vegetables
1 1/2 cups cauliflower florets
1 1/2 cups trimmed green beans

Sauce
1 Tbsp light, soft tub margarine
1 Tbsp unbleached white flour
1/2 cup evaporated nonfat milk
1 1/2 oz crumbled bleu cheese
2 tsp Dijon mustard

Exchanges	
2 Vegetable	
1/2 Fat	
Calories	72
Calories from Fat	27
Total Fat	3 g
Saturated Fat	1.3 g
Cholesterol	5 mg
Sodium	189 mg
Total Carbohydrate	8 g
Dietary Fiber	2 g
Sugars	3 g
Protein	4 g

1. Steam the cauliflower over boiling water on a steamer rack for 5 minutes. Add the green beans and steam for an additional 2–3 minutes. Remove from heat.

2. Meanwhile, make the sauce. In a large skillet, heat the margarine. Add the flour and stir until smooth. Add the milk and cook until bubbly. Add the cheese and mustard. Toss in the cooked vegetables and serve.

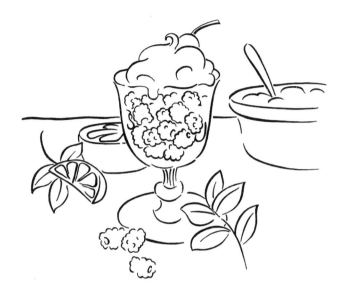

SWEET ENDINGS

Nothing completes a meal like dessert, but who has the time to make dessert and dinner? Fortunately, preparing dessert does not have to be a complicated process. In this chapter, simple ingredients are turned into spectacular creations.

You'll get the best results with some of the fruit desserts if you use fresh fruit. Canned or frozen fruit does not hold up as well or taste as good. Buying fruits when they are in season will ensure the best-tasting desserts.

So, go ahead—indulge in these healthy sweet endings!

BERRIES WITH ITALIAN CREAM

HOT FRUIT COMPOTE

PUMPKIN MOUSSE

POACHED CINNAMON ORANGES

CHOCOLATE SPICE PUDDING

BLUEBERRIES CHANTILLY

GLAZED FRUIT

STOVETOP APPLE-RICE PUDDING

Berries with Italian Cream

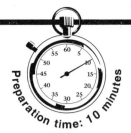
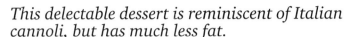

Preparation time: 10 minutes

Total Servings: 6
Serving Size: 1/2 cup

This delectable dessert is reminiscent of Italian cannoli, but has much less fat.

3 cups sliced fresh strawberries or raspberries
1 tsp sugar
1 15-oz carton fat-free ricotta cheese
1 Tbsp Grand Marnier
1 tsp vanilla
1 1/2 tsp grated orange peel

Exchanges	
1 Fruit	
1 Very Lean Meat	
Calories	88
Calories from Fat	3
Total Fat	0 g
Saturated Fat	0 g
Cholesterol	23 mg
Sodium	58 mg
Total Carbohydrate	11 g
Dietary Fiber	2 g
Sugars	7 g
Protein	10 g

1. In a medium bowl, mix together the berries and the sugar. Set aside.

2. With an electric beater, beat together the remaining ingredients until light and fluffy.

3. Divide berries among dessert dishes. Top each serving with a portion of the cream.

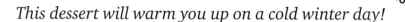

Hot Fruit Compote

Total Servings: 6
Serving Size: 1/2 cup

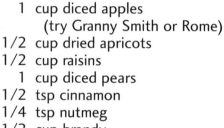

This dessert will warm you up on a cold winter day!

1 cup diced apples
　(try Granny Smith or Rome)
1/2 cup dried apricots
1/2 cup raisins
1 cup diced pears
1/2 tsp cinnamon
1/4 tsp nutmeg
1/2 cup brandy
2 Tbsp lemon juice
2 tsp honey

Exchanges	
1 1/2 Fruit	
Calories	111
Calories from Fat	3
Total Fat	0 g
Saturated Fat	0 g
Cholesterol	0 mg
Sodium	4 mg
Total Carbohydrate	25 g
Dietary Fiber	3 g
Sugars	19 g
Protein	1 g

Combine all ingredients and mix well. Place in a casserole dish and bake at 350°F for 20 minutes until the fruit is soft.

Pumpkin Mousse

Total Servings: 6
Serving Size: 1/2 cup

Preparation time: 6 minutes

*Pumpkin is a wonderful source of vitamin A. Be sure
to include this nutritious vegetable in desserts throughout the year,
not just during the holidays.*

2 cups canned pumpkin (not pumpkin
   pie filling)
1 Tbsp honey
2 tsp cinnamon
2 tsp grated lemon peel
1 cup fat-free ricotta cheese

Exchanges	
1/2 Carbohydrate	
Calories	57
Calories from Fat	1
Total Fat	0 g
Saturated Fat	0.1 g
Cholesterol	13 mg
Sodium	36 mg
Total Carbohydrate	9 g
Dietary Fiber	2 g
Sugars	6 g
Protein	6 g

In a medium bowl, combine the pumpkin, honey, cinnamon, and
lemon peel. Mix well. Fold in the ricotta cheese. Refrigerate for 1
hour and serve.

Poached Cinnamon Oranges

Total Servings: 6
Serving Size: 1/2 cup

Jazz up plain citrus with a warm cinnamon syrup.
(If you use unsweetened grape juice, the nutrient analysis in parentheses applies.)

3 large oranges, peeled and
   sliced into 1/2-inch rounds
2 cups red wine or unsweetened
   grape juice
1 Tbsp honey
2 cinnamon sticks
2 tsp vanilla
2 tsp grated orange peel

Exchanges	
1 (2) Fruit	
Calories	83 (111)
Calories from Fat	1 (2)
Total Fat	0 g (0 g)
Saturated Fat	0 g (0 g)
Cholesterol	0 g (0 g)
Sodium	2 mg (3 mg)
Total Carbohydrate	16 g (28 g)
Dietary Fiber	2 g (3 g)
Sugars	12 g (24 g)
Protein	1 g (1 g)

1. Prepare the oranges and set aside.

2. In a medium saucepan over medium heat, combine the wine or juice, honey, and cinnamon sticks. Bring to a boil. Reduce the heat and cook for 15 minutes.

3. Remove from the heat and add the vanilla and orange peel. Pour over the oranges in a bowl and refrigerate 1 hour. Serve.

Chocolate Spice Pudding

Total Servings: 6
Serving Size: 1/2 cup

Chocolate lovers, rejoice! This spicy pudding tastes
like the pudding from your childhood (but it's much healthier).

Preparation time: 10 minutes

1/3	cup unsweetened cocoa powder
1/4	cup sugar
1	Tbsp cornstarch or arrowroot powder
1/2	tsp ginger
1/4	tsp allspice
1	tsp cinnamon
3	cups evaporated nonfat milk
1	egg yolk, slightly beaten
3	tsp vanilla

Exchanges

1 Fat-Free Milk

1 Carbohydrate

Calories...................... 157
  Calories from Fat...... 16
Total Fat..................... 2 g
  Saturated Fat........... 1 g
Cholesterol........... 40 mg
Sodium................ 149 mg
Total Carbohydrate 27 g
  Dietary Fiber............. 1 g
  Sugars...................... 20 g
Protein .... 11 g

1. Mix first six ingredients in a saucepan. Stir in the milk and egg yolk. Cook until the mixture thickens, stirring constantly.

2. Remove from heat and add vanilla. Pour into six custard dishes. Chill and serve.

Blueberries Chantilly

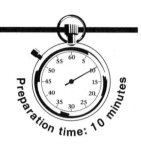

Total Servings: 6
Serving Size: 1/2 cup fruit with 1/4 cup topping

Clouds of light sour cream and cream cheese surround plump, juicy blueberries.

2	cups fresh blueberries
1	cup fresh raspberries
1	cup fat-free sour cream
1/2	cup fat-free cream cheese
1	Tbsp orange juice
1	Tbsp honey
1	tsp cinnamon
2	tsp orange peel

Exchanges
1 1/2 Carbohydrate

Calories	105
Calories from Fat	3
Total Fat	0 g
Saturated Fat	0 g
Cholesterol	5 mg
Sodium	171 mg
Total Carbohydrate	21 g
Dietary Fiber	3 g
Sugars	11 g
Protein	5 g

Place the blueberries and raspberries in a large bowl. With electric beaters, whip together the sour cream, cream cheese, orange juice, honey, and cinnamon until light and fluffy. Spread over the top of the berries. Garnish with orange peel and serve.

Diabetic Meals in 30 Minutes—Or Less!

Glazed Fruit

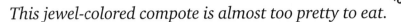

Total Servings: 6
Serving Size: 1/2 cup

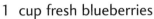

This jewel-colored compote is almost too pretty to eat.

1 cup fresh blueberries
1 cup sliced strawberries
1 cup sliced peaches
1/4 cup low-sugar blackberry preserves
1/4 cup low-sugar orange marmalade
2 Tbsp lemon juice
1 tsp grated lemon peel

Exchanges	
1 Fruit	
Calories	58
Calories from Fat	2
Total Fat	0 g
Saturated Fat	0 g
Cholesterol	0 mg
Sodium	12 mg
Total Carbohydrate	14 g
Dietary Fiber	2 g
Sugars	8 g
Protein	0 g

1. Grouping together in rows, place the fruit in a large glass bowl.

2. In two separate small saucepans, heat each jam with one half of the lemon juice and lemon peel until it boils.

3. Pour each melted jam on one half of the fruit. Serve.

Stovetop Apple-Rice Pudding

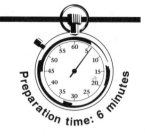

Total Servings: 6
Serving Size: 1/2 cup

Apple pie spice and applesauce make this a delicious variation of traditional rice pudding.

Pudding

        2 cups evaporated nonfat milk
        1 8-oz jar unsweetened applesauce
    1/2 cup raisins
        2 Tbsp fructose
        1 tsp apple pie spice
1 1/2 cups quick-cooking rice

Garnish

        Apple pie spice

Exchanges	
1 1/2 Starch	
1 Fruit	
1/2 Fat-Free Milk	
Calories	222
Calories from Fat	3
Total Fat	0 g
Saturated Fat	0 g
Cholesterol	3 mg
Sodium	102 mg
Total Carbohydrate	46 g
Dietary Fiber	1 g
Sugars	22 g
Protein	9 g

1. In a saucepan, combine the milk, applesauce, raisins, fructose, and apple pie spice. Bring to a boil, then stir in the rice.

2. Cover and simmer for about 10–15 minutes until liquid is absorbed. Spoon into dessert dishes and dust with apple pie spice. Serve warm or cold.

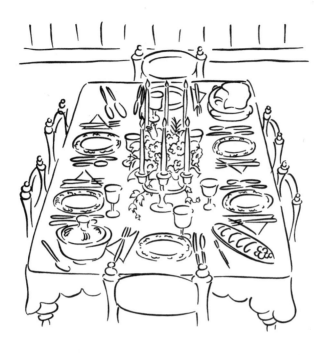

Complete Menus
for
Every Day
and
Entertaining

When you need a complete menu in a hurry, look no further than these appetizing theme menus—suitable for every day and for entertaining. Each menu serves six people. Shopping lists are provided, as well as a "countdown" timetable that shows you the order in which to prepare your food, so all of your meal will be ready to eat at the same time!

ROMANTIC DINING

LAZY SUNDAY BRUNCH

60
55   5

COUNTRY FRENCH DINNER

50   10

45   15

40   WARM SUMMER EVENING   20

35   25

30

DINNER ITALIANO

Romantic Dining

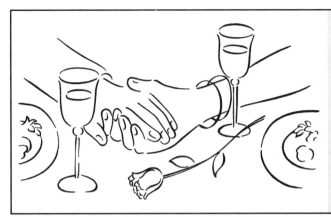

Menu

*Broiled Salmon with
  Roasted Red Pepper
  Sauce*

Herbed Potatoes

*Green Beans with
  Shiitake Mushrooms*

Fresh Raspberries

Shopping List

1 1/2 lb salmon fillets

Olive oil

Lemon juice

1 12-oz jar roasted red
  peppers

Evaporated nonfat milk

Dried or fresh oregano

Onions

1 small shallot

1 1/2 lb small red
  potatoes

1 lb fresh green beans

1/2 lb fresh shiitake
  mushrooms

Lite soy sauce

Low-fat, reduced-
  sodium chicken
  broth

1 1/2 pints raspberries

Rosemary

Thyme

Paprika

White wine

Countdown

1. Prepare the Herb Potatoes.
2. While the Herb Potatoes are baking, prepare the Roasted Red Pepper Sauce. Set sauce aside in a saucepot.
3. Wash the raspberries, place in individual glass dessert dishes, and place the dishes in the refrigerator.
4. Prepare the salmon, but do not broil yet.
5. Prepare the Green Beans with Shiitake Mushrooms.
6. Remove the potatoes from the oven. Place the salmon steaks under the broiler.
7. Heat the Roasted Red Pepper Sauce.
8. Place the salmon, green beans, and potatoes on a plate and serve.
9. Serve fresh raspberries for dessert!

Broiled Salmon with Roasted Red Pepper Sauce

Total Servings: 6
Serving Size: 3 oz salmon with 2–3 Tbsp sauce

Preparation time: 15 minutes

Salmon

     2 tsp olive oil
     2 Tbsp fresh lemon juice
1 1/2 lb salmon fillets

Sauce

     2 tsp olive oil
     1 medium onion, minced
     1 12-oz jar roasted red peppers,
         drained and chopped
     3 Tbsp evaporated nonfat milk
     2 tsp fresh minced oregano (or 1 tsp
         dried)
         Fresh ground pepper and salt to taste

Exchanges
1 Vegetable
3 Lean Meat
1 Fat

Calories	240
Calories from Fat	116
Total Fat	13 g
Saturated Fat	2 g
Cholesterol	77 mg
Sodium	168 mg
Total Carbohydrate	5 g
Dietary Fiber	1 g
Sugars	3 g
Protein	25 g

1. Combine the lemon juice and olive oil and brush over the salmon. Let the salmon sit at room temperature for 10 minutes.

2. To make the sauce, heat the oil in a small skillet over medium-high heat. Add the onion and sauté for 5 minutes.

3. In a blender, puree the onions with the roasted red peppers. Add the evaporated milk and oregano. Season with pepper and mix well.

4. Place the salmon on a broiler rack set 6 inches from the heat source. Broil the salmon for about 10 minutes until the salmon is tender.

5. Heat the sauce in a small saucepan. To serve, place a small pool of sauce on a dinner plate. Top with a 3-oz salmon fillet. Spoon some sauce on top. Repeat with all fillets.

Herbed Potatoes

Total Servings: 6
Serving Size: 1/2 cup

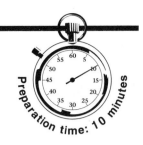

Preparation time: 10 minutes

1 1/2 lb small red potatoes
1 1/2 tsp olive oil
   6 sprigs rosemary
   6 sprigs thyme
   2 Tbsp white wine
2 1/2 tsp paprika

Exchanges	
1 1/2 Starch	
Calories	110
Calories from Fat	11
Total Fat	1 g
Saturated Fat	0 g
Cholesterol	0 mg
Sodium	6 mg
Total Carbohydrate	23 g
Dietary Fiber	2 g
Sugars	2 g
Protein	2 g

1. Preheat the oven to 400°F. Wash and scrub the potatoes. Cut each potato in half.

2. Place about 1/2 cup of potatoes on six squares of foil large enough to fold over. Divide the olive oil, herbs, wine, and paprika evenly over each packet. Seal the packets and place in the oven.

3. Bake for 30 minutes. Let cool for 5 minutes. Place a packet on each plate and let each person carefully open the packet.

Green Beans with Shiitake Mushrooms

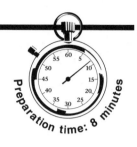

Total Servings: 6
Serving Size: 1/2 cup

3 Tbsp	low-fat, reduced-sodium chicken broth
1	small shallot, minced
1 lb	trimmed green beans, cut into 1-inch lengths
1/2 lb	sliced and stemmed shiitake mushrooms
2 Tbsp	lite soy sauce

Exchanges
2 Vegetable

Calories	41
Calories from Fat	3
Total Fat	0 g
Saturated Fat	0 g
Cholesterol	0 mg
Sodium	208 mg
Total Carbohydrate	9 g
Dietary Fiber	3 g
Sugars	4 g
Protein	2 g

1. In a skillet over medium heat, heat the broth. Add the shallot and sauté for 3 minutes.

2. Add the green beans and shiitake mushrooms. Stir-fry for 5 minutes. Add the soy sauce. Cover and steam for 2 minutes.

Diabetic Meals in 30 Minutes—Or Less!

LAZY SUNDAY BRUNCH

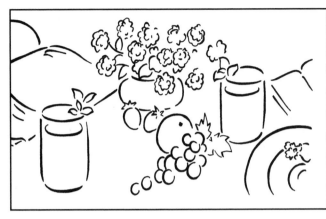

MENU

*Scrambled Eggs in
  Crisp Potato Skins*

Spicy Turkey Sausages

Whole-Grain Toast

Banana Mint Slushes

SHOPPING LIST

Eggs or egg substitutes

3 large baking
  potatoes

Olive oil

Paprika

1 red pepper

1 green pepper

Reduced-fat or fat-free
  cream cheese

Cilantro

Parsley

Fennel seeds

Crushed red pepper
  flakes

Cumin

Cloves

1 lb lean ground
  turkey

Whole-grain bread

2 bananas

Mint

Vanilla extract

Nonfat milk

COUNTDOWN

1. Prepare the turkey sausage mixture the night before to let the flavors blend.
2. The next day, prepare the potato skins.
3. Slice the whole-grain bread, if not already sliced.
4. Cook the sausages and keep warm.
5. Cook the eggs and place in the cooked potato shells.
6. While toasting whole-grain bread, prepare the banana mint slushes.
7. Place the eggs, sausages, and bread on plates. Pour the slushes in a pitcher. Serve.

Scrambled Eggs in Crisp Potato Skins

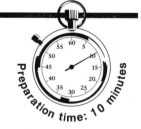

Total Servings: 6
Serving Size: 2 eggs with 1/2 large baked potato skin

Shells

    3 large cooked baking potatoes, cut in
       half and scooped out (leave a
       1-inch shell)
1 1/2 tsp olive oil
      Paprika

Eggs

      Nonstick cooking spray
1/2 cup each diced red and green pepper
 12 egg substitutes, beaten
  2 Tbsp reduced-fat or fat-free cream
      cheese

Exchanges	
1 Starch	
2 Very Lean Meat	
Calories	153
Calories from Fat	18
Total Fat	2 g
Saturated Fat	1 g
Cholesterol	3 mg
Sodium	241 mg
Total Carbohydrate	18 g
Dietary Fiber	1 g
Sugars	3 g
Protein	15 g

1. Preheat the oven to 400°F. Place the scooped-out potato skins on a baking sheet. Brush the skins with oil. Dust each shell with paprika. Bake in the oven for 20 minutes.

2. To prepare the eggs, place a nonstick skillet over medium heat and spray the skillet lightly with cooking spray. Add the peppers and sauté for 5 minutes.

3. Add the eggs and cook about 5 minutes until eggs are set. Add the cream cheese and blend in well.

4. To serve, pile the eggs into the potato shells and dust with more paprika.

Spicy Turkey Sausages

Total Servings: 6
Serving Size: 2 oz

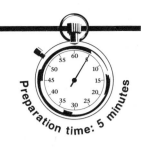

Preparation time: 5 minutes

1/2 cup finely minced cilantro
1/2 cup finely minced parsley
2 tsp fennel seeds
1/4 tsp cumin
1/4 tsp cloves
1 tsp crushed red pepper flakes
Fresh ground pepper and salt to taste
1 lb lean ground turkey (your butcher can grind this for you)

Exchanges	
2 Very Lean Meat	
Calories	84
Calories from Fat	4
Total Fat	0 g
Saturated Fat	0 g
Cholesterol	50 mg
Sodium	58 mg
Total Carbohydrate	0 g
Dietary Fiber	0 g
Sugars	0 g
Protein	18 g

1. Combine all ingredients in a food processor or mix together very well by hand.

2. Let the turkey mixture chill for several hours. Then form the mixture into patties.

3. In a nonstick skillet, cook the patties on each side for 3–4 minutes, until the turkey is cooked through.

Banana Mint Slushes

Total Servings: 6
Serving Size: 1/2 cup

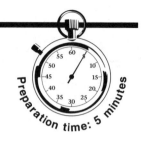

Preparation time: 5 minutes

 2 bananas
10 mint leaves
 2 tsp vanilla extract
 3 cups nonfat milk
 1 cup ice cubes

Exchanges		
1/2 Fruit		
1/2 Fat-Free Milk		
Calories		76
Calories from Fat		3
Total Fat		0 g
Saturated Fat		0 g
Cholesterol		2 mg
Sodium		63 mg
Total Carbohydrate		14 g
Dietary Fiber		1 g
Sugars		11 g
Protein		5 g

Place the bananas in a blender and puree. Add the remaining ingredients and blend well. Serve from a tall pitcher in frosty glasses.

COUNTRY FRENCH DINNER

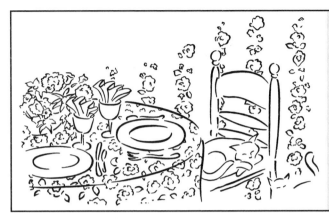

MENU

*Chicken with Tarragon
and Mushrooms*

Carrots with Fennel

Roasted Potatoes

Macédoine of Fruit

SHOPPING LIST

3 whole chicken
   breasts

Tarragon

1 lb sliced mushrooms

Dry white wine

3 shallots

3 cups small carrots

Port wine

Fennel seeds

Olive oil

1 lb small red potatoes

2 medium apples

2 bananas

Red grapes

1 orange

Orange liqueur

Lemon juice

COUNTDOWN

1. Prepare the Macédoine of Fruit and set in the refrigerator until time for dessert.
2. Drizzle red potatoes with a little olive oil and place in the oven to roast for 30 minutes.
3. Prepare the carrots.
4. Prepare the chicken.
5. Remove the potatoes from the oven and place on plates with the chicken and carrot packets.
6. Serve dessert.

Chicken with Tarragon and Mushrooms

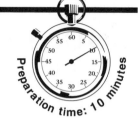

Total Servings: 6
Serving Size: 3–4 oz chicken with sauce

3 whole chicken breasts, halved, boned, and skinned
6 sprigs tarragon
3 shallots, minced
1/4 cup dry white wine
1 lb sliced mushrooms
    Fresh ground pepper and salt to taste

Exchanges	
1 Vegetable	
4 Very Lean Meat	
Calories	163
Calories from Fat	30
Total Fat	3 g
Saturated Fat	1 g
Cholesterol	73 mg
Sodium	89 mg
Total Carbohydrate	4 g
Dietary Fiber	1 g
Sugars	1 g
Protein	28 g

1. Preheat the oven to 350°F. Tear aluminum foil into six squares large enough to seal the chicken.

2. Place a chicken breast on each foil piece. Place the remaining ingredients on top of each breast, dividing evenly. Fold the foil over to seal. Place the chicken packets in the oven and bake for about 15 minutes.

3. Place the packets on individual plates and let each person carefully open the packet.

Diabetic Meals in 30 Minutes—Or Less!

Carrots with Fennel

Total Servings: 6
Serving Size: 1/2 cup

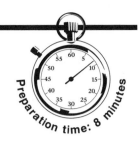

Preparation time: 8 minutes

3 cups baby carrots
3 Tbsp port wine
1 Tbsp fennel seeds
1 Tbsp olive oil
Fresh ground pepper and salt to taste

Exchanges	
2 Vegetable	
1/2 Fat	
Calories	60
Calories from Fat	22
Total Fat	2 g
Saturated Fat	0 g
Cholesterol	0 mg
Sodium	72 mg
Total Carbohydrate	8 g
Dietary Fiber	3 g
Sugars	3 g
Protein	1 g

1. Preheat the oven to 350°F. Tear aluminum foil into six pieces large enough to seal the carrots.

2. Divide all ingredients evenly among all six pieces of foil. Crimp to seal. Place the packets in the oven and bake for 15 minutes, until carrots are tender.

3. Place the packets on individual plates and let each person carefully open the packet.

Macédoine of Fruit

Total Servings: 6
Serving Size: 1/2 cup

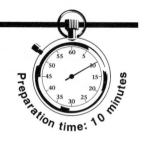

Preparation time: 10 minutes

2 medium apples, unpeeled and thinly sliced
2 bananas, thinly sliced
1 cup red grapes
1 orange, peeled and sliced
1 Tbsp orange liqueur
2 Tbsp lemon juice

Exchanges	
1 1/2 Fruit	
Calories	102
Calories from Fat	5
Total Fat	1 g
Saturated Fat	0 g
Cholesterol	0 mg
Sodium	2 mg
Total Carbohydrate	25 g
Dietary Fiber	3 g
Sugars	19 g
Protein	1 g

Combine all ingredients in a large glass bowl. Toss to mix well. Refrigerate and serve chilled.

WARM SUMMER EVENING

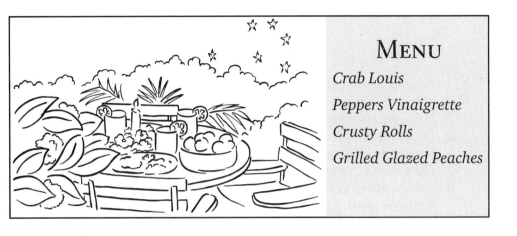

MENU

Crab Louis

Peppers Vinaigrette

Crusty Rolls

Grilled Glazed Peaches

SHOPPING LIST

1 1/2 lb lump crabmeat

Reduced-fat mayonnaise

Evaporated nonfat milk

Hot chili sauce

Lemon juice

Scallions

Romaine lettuce

1 red pepper

1 yellow pepper

2 green peppers

Red wine vinegar

Fresh chives

Olive oil

Whole-grain rolls

3 large peaches

Low-calorie margarine

Orange juice

Sugar

COUNTDOWN

1. Prepare the peppers and chill.
2. Prepare the Crab Louis and place on a platter.
3. Set out the rolls.
4. Remove the peppers from the refrigerator and serve with the Crab Louis and rolls.
5. Grill the peaches and eat.

Crab Louis

Total Servings: 6
Serving Size: 3 oz

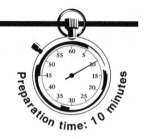

1 1/2 lb lump crabmeat
1/2 cup reduced-fat mayonnaise
2 Tbsp evaporated nonfat milk
2 Tbsp hot chili sauce
1 Tbsp lemon juice
2 Tbsp diced green pepper
3 Tbsp minced scallions
    Romaine lettuce leaves

Exchanges	
1/2 Starch	
3 Very Lean Meat	
Calories	143
Calories from Fat	27
Total Fat	3 g
Saturated Fat	0 g
Cholesterol	96 mg
Sodium	529 mg
Total Carbohydrate	8 g
Dietary Fiber	0 g
Sugars	5 g
Protein	20 g

Combine all ingredients. Set crabmeat on top of romaine lettuce leaves and serve.

Peppers Vinaigrette

Total Servings: 6
Serving Size: 1/2 cup

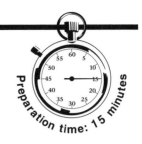

1 each small green, yellow, and red peppers, thinly sliced
2 Tbsp olive oil
1/4 cup red wine vinegar
1 tsp sugar
2 Tbsp minced chives
Fresh ground pepper and salt to taste

Exchanges	
1 Vegetable	
1 Fat	
Calories	60
Calories from Fat	41
Total Fat	5 g
Saturated Fat	1 g
Cholesterol	0 mg
Sodium	25 mg
Total Carbohydrate	5 g
Dietary Fiber	1 g
Sugars	3 g
Protein	1 g

1. In a pot of boiling water, add the peppers and cook for 2 minutes. Drain and plunge in ice water. Drain again.

2. In a blender, blend together the remaining ingredients. Pour over the peppers and mix well. Serve.

Grilled Glazed Peaches

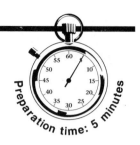

Total Servings: 6
Serving Size: 1/2 large peach

1/4 cup light, soft tub margarine
2 Tbsp orange juice
3 large peaches, pitted and halved, unpeeled

Exchanges	
1/2 Fruit	
1/2 Fat	
Calories	60
Calories from Fat	29
Total Fat	3 g
Saturated Fat	0.3 g
Cholesterol	0 mg
Sodium	60 mg
Total Carbohydrate	8 g
Dietary Fiber	1 g
Sugars	7 g
Protein	1 g

1. Prepare a hot grill. In a separate pan, melt the margarine and orange juice until syrupy.

2. Place the peaches, cut side down, on an oiled rack 6 inches from the heat source. Brush the syrup over the peaches. Grill the peaches about 10 minutes, turning and basting frequently, until the peaches are hot and glazed. Remove from the grill and serve.

Diabetic Meals in 30 Minutes—Or Less!

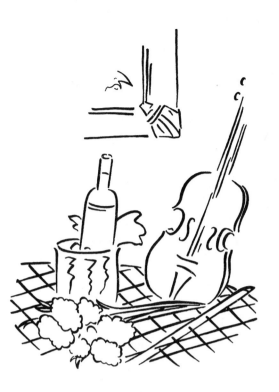

DINNER ITALIANO

SHOPPING LIST

1 lb rigatoni

3/4 lb chicken breasts

1 onion

1 green pepper

1 15-oz jar marinara sauce

4 small zucchini

Parmesan cheese

6 cups salad greens

3 cups plain nonfat yogurt

1 banana

1 cup green grapes

1 cup strawberries

Grape-Nuts® cereal

2 eggs or egg substitute

Unbleached white flour

Olive oil

Balsamic vinegar

Vanilla extract

Dried basil

Dried oregano

Garlic powder

Paprika

Dijon mustard

Fresh garlic

Shallots

Fructose

COUNTDOWN

1. Prepare the Layered Vanilla Yogurt Parfaits and refrigerate until time for dessert.
2. Prepare the salad dressing. Refrigerate.
3. Wash the salad greens. Place in a salad bowl. Cover and refrigerate.
4. Slice the zucchini. Coat with the Parmesan mixture and place on a cookie sheet. Place the cookie sheet in the refrigerator and let the coating adhere to the zucchini for 15 minutes before baking.
5. Prepare the dessert and refrigerate.
6. Boil the rigatoni.
7. Prepare the sauce for the rigatoni.
8. Place the zucchini in the oven and bake for 7 minutes.
9. Pour sauce over pasta and place in serving bowl.
10. Take zucchini out of the oven and place in serving bowl.
11. Shake dressing, pour over greens, and toss.
12. Serve dinner.
13. Serve dessert.

Chicken Rigatoni

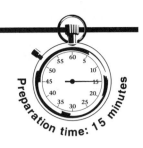

Preparation time: 15 minutes

Total Servings: 6
Serving Size: 2 oz chicken with 1 cup pasta

1 Tbsp olive oil
3/4 lb boneless, skinless chicken breasts, cubed
1 medium onion, chopped
1 green pepper, seeded, cored, and cut into matchstick strips
1 15-oz jar marinara sauce
Fresh ground pepper to taste
6 cups cooked rigatoni pasta

Exchanges	
2 Vegetable	
2 Lean Meat	
Calories	312
Calories from Fat	62
Total Fat	7 g
Saturated Fat	2 g
Cholesterol	35 mg
Sodium	284 mg
Total Carbohydrate	41 g
Dietary Fiber	4 g
Sugars	6 g
Protein	19 g

1. To prepare the sauce, heat the oil in a large skillet over medium heat. Add the chicken and sauté until chicken is no longer pink. Remove from the skillet.

2. In the remaining pan juices, sauté the onion and pepper. Add the cooked chicken to the skillet and add the marinara sauce. Grind in pepper.

3. Let the sauce simmer for about 5 minutes. Pour over the rigatoni and serve.

Oven-Baked Parmesan Zucchini

Total Servings: 6
Serving Size: 1/2 cup

4 small zucchini, scrubbed and
      diagonally sliced about 1/2 inch
      thick
2 eggs or egg substitutes, beaten
2 Tbsp unbleached white flour
3 Tbsp Parmesan cheese
1 tsp dried oregano
1/2 tsp dried basil
1 tsp paprika
1/2 tsp garlic powder
1 Tbsp olive oil

Exchanges	
1 Vegetable	
1/2 Fat	
Calories	51
Calories from Fat	25
Total Fat	3 g
Saturated Fat	1 g
Cholesterol	1 mg
Sodium	57 mg
Total Carbohydrate	4 g
Dietary Fiber	1 g
Sugars	2 g
Protein	3 g

1. Preheat the oven to 350°F. Dip each zucchini slice into the beaten egg.

2. In a large plastic zip-top bag, combine the remaining ingredients except the oil. Shake the mixture well. Add the zucchini slices and shake well.

3. Place the zucchini slices on a nonstick cookie sheet. Drizzle the zucchini slices with the olive oil.

4. Bake for 7–8 minutes until zucchini is golden brown.

Balsamic Vinaigrette

Total Servings: 8
Serving Size: 2 Tbsp

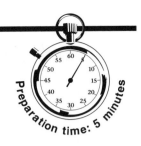

1/2 cup balsamic vinegar
2 tsp minced garlic
3 tsp Dijon mustard
1 Tbsp olive oil
1/4 cup minced shallots
Fresh ground pepper and salt to taste

Exchanges	
1/2 Fat	
Calories	23
Calories from Fat	16
Total Fat	2 g
Saturated Fat	0 g
Cholesterol	0 mg
Sodium	42 mg
Total Carbohydrate	2 g
Dietary Fiber	0 g
Sugars	1 g
Protein	0 g

In a small bowl, whisk together all ingredients. Serve over salad greens. You can store this dressing in the refrigerator for up to 2 weeks.

Layered Vanilla Yogurt Parfaits

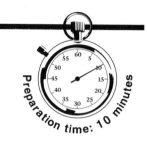

Total Servings: 6
Serving Size: 1/2 cup yogurt with 1/2 cup fruit

3 cups plain nonfat yogurt
2 tsp vanilla extract
3 tsp fructose
1 banana, sliced
1 cup halved green grapes
1 cup sliced strawberries
1/4 cup Grape-Nuts® cereal

Exchanges	
1 Fruit	
1/2 Fat-Free Milk	
Calories	126
Calories from Fat	3
Total Fat	0 g
Saturated Fat	0 g
Cholesterol	3 mg
Sodium	129 mg
Total Carbohydrate	25 g
Dietary Fiber	2 g
Sugars	19 g
Protein	8 g

1. In a small bowl, combine the yogurt, vanilla, and fructose. Place a bottom layer of the yogurt mixture in parfait, wine, or champagne glasses.

2. In another bowl, combine the fruits. Add a layer of fruit on top of the yogurt. Continue layering the yogurt and fruit until each glass has three layers, ending with yogurt.

3. Top each parfait with a sprinkle of Grape-Nuts® cereal. Chill until ready to serve.

Diabetic Meals in 30 Minutes—Or Less!

INDEX

Alphabetical List of Recipes

Subject Index

Appetizers (see *Dips*)

Asian Dishes

Beans

Vegetables—*continued*

Other Titles Available from the American Diabetes Association

GUIDE TO HEALTHY RESTAURANT EATING, 3RD ED.

By Hope S. Warshaw, MMSc, RD, CDE, BC-ADM

Eat out without guilt or sacrifice! Newly updated, this bestselling guide features more than 5,000 menu items for over 60 restaurant chains. This is the most comprehensive guide to restaurant nutrition for people with diabetes who like to eat out.

Order #4819-03; $17.95 US

TYPE 2 DIABETES FOR BEGINNERS

By Phyllis Barrier, MS, RD, CDE

If you've recently been diagnosed with type 2 diabetes, this book is the introduction you need for staying healthy. You'll get the straight facts about living with type 2 diabetes and straight answers to your questions about the disease.

Order #4877-01; $14.95 US

THE DIABETES CARBOHYDRATE & FAT GRAM GUIDE, 3RD ED.

By Lea Ann Holzmeister, RD, CDE

This guide is now better than ever. Registered dietitian Lea Ann Holzmeister has gone back to the drawing board and put together complete nutritional information, including carbs, fat, calories, and more for nearly 7,000 listings. This new edition now features charts for fast foods and prepackaged meals.

Order #4708-03; $14.95 US

AMERICAN DIABETES ASSOCIATION COMPLETE GUIDE TO DIABETES, 4TH ED.

By the American Diabetes Association

The world's largest collection of diabetes self-care tips, techniques, and tricks you can use to solve diabetes-related troubles just got bigger and better!

Order #4809-04; $29.95 US

To order these and other great American Diabetes Association titles, call 1-800-232-6733 or visit http://store.diabetes.org. American Diabetes Association titles are also available in bookstores nationwide.

About the American Diabetes Association

The American Diabetes Association is the nation's leading voluntary health organization supporting diabetes research, information, and advocacy. Its mission is to prevent and cure diabetes and to improve the lives of all people affected by diabetes. The American Diabetes Association is the leading publisher of comprehensive diabetes information. Its huge library of practical and authoritative books for people with diabetes covers every aspect of self-care—cooking and nutrition, fitness, weight control, medications, complications, emotional issues, and general self-care.

To order American Diabetes Association books: Call 1-800-232-6733 or log on to http://store.diabetes.org

To join the American Diabetes Association: Call 1-800-806-7801 or log on to www.diabetes.org/membership

For more information about diabetes or ADA programs and services: Call 1-800-342-2383. E-mail: AskADA@diabetes.org or log on to www.diabetes.org

To locate an ADA/NCQA Recognized Provider of quality diabetes care in your area: www.ncqa.org/dprp

To find an ADA Recognized Education Program in your area: Call 1-800-342-2383. www.diabetes.org/for-health-professionals-and-scientists/recognition/edrecognition.jsp

To join the fight to increase funding for diabetes research, end discrimination, and improve insurance coverage: Call 1-800-342-2383. www.diabetes.org/advocacy-and-legalresources/advocacy.jsp

To find out how you can get involved with the programs in your community: Call 1-800-342-2383. See below for program Web addresses.

American Diabetes Month: educational activities aimed at those diagnosed with diabetes—month of November. www.diabetes.org/communityprograms-and-localevents/americandiabetesmonth.jsp

American Diabetes Alert: annual public awareness campaign to find the undiagnosed—held the fourth Tuesday in March. www.diabetes.org/communityprograms-and-localevents/americandiabetesalert.jsp

The Diabetes Assistance & Resources Program (DAR): diabetes awareness program targeted to the Latino community. www.diabetes.org/communityprograms-and-localevents/latinos.jsp

African American Program: diabetes awareness program targeted to the African American community. www.diabetes.org/communityprograms-and-localevents/africanamericans.jsp

Awakening the Spirit: Pathways to Diabetes Prevention & Control: diabetes awareness program targeted to the Native American community. www.diabetes.org/communityprograms-and-localevents/nativeamericans.jsp

To find out about an important research project regarding type 2 diabetes: www.diabetes.org/diabetes-research/research-home.jsp

To obtain information on making a planned gift or charitable bequest: Call 1-888-700-7029. www.wpg.cc/stl/CDA/homepage/1,1006,509,00.html

To make a donation or memorial contribution: Call 1-800-342-2383. www.diabetes.org/support-the-cause/make-a-donation.jsp